DON'T
LOSE
SIGHT

DON'T LOSE SIGHT

Vanity, incompetence, and my ill-fated left eye

GENEVIEVE A. CHORNENKI

IGUANA

Published by Iguana Books
720 Bathurst Street, Suite 303
Toronto, ON M5S 2R4

Publisher: Meghan Behse
Cover and text designer: Tania Craan
Cover images: (island) Jorik Kleen, Groningen/Unsplash,
    (clouds) Romello Williams/Unsplash
Page 13: Drew Brown/Unsplash
Page 63: David Clode/Unsplash
Page 97: Chuttersnap/Unsplash
Author photo: (leaf) Drew Graham/Unsplash,
    (author headshot) Bo Huang Photography

ISBN 978-1-77180-480-6 (paperback)
ISBN 978-1-77180-481-3 (epub)

This is an original print edition of *Don't Lose Sight: Vanity, incompetence, and my ill-fated left eye.*

*For my left eye whom,
together with the right, I worship and glorify.*

I am learning to see. Yes, I am beginning. It's still going badly.
But I intend to make the most of my time.
—RAINER MARIA RILKE,
The Notebooks of Malte Laurids Brigge

CONTENTS
. . . .

PREFACE

They need not be Damascus raptures, our moments of soul.
    —Christian Wiman

I spy with both my eyes.

A gigantic rose in the deepest of purples, daubed here and there with celadon and washed with blue-grey. A red cabbage on my cutting board.

One at a time I snap off its outer petals, then briskly bifurcate the brassica with a sharp knife. Layered treasures line its interior. Waves of garnet. Veins of opal. Sparks of amethyst. Tourmaline. I reduce these cabbage-gems to shreds and mound them in a pot. It's an ordinary stainless steel pot from Ikea, but it brims with wonder, and I with childish delight.

"William. Come and see!" My husband obliges and together we contemplate the contents of the pot. "Man," I say. "Is that not amazing?"

Forget seeing Machu Picchu. This meal-in-the-making is my peak pleasure. Cut red cabbage calls up reverence and awe. How come? Because, Joni, I do know what I've got before it's gone. Because my ability to see this cabbage—all of it, in depth, without distortion—was in peril. Because I got lucky, and I know it.

Something happened. And then something else and then something more. Many things, seen and unseen, beginning with my left eye.

PART I

Nothing Is Obvious to the Uninformed

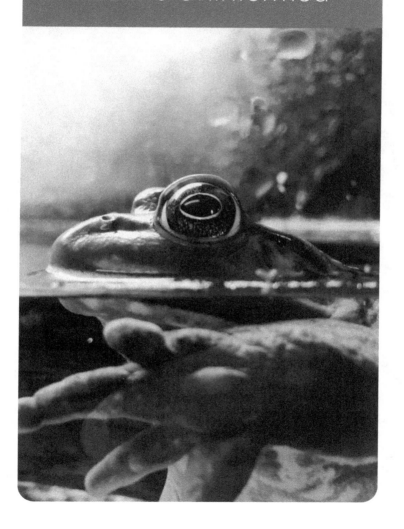

CHAPTER 1

Appearances
....

"You coming?" My roommate, Daphne, calls from the door of our apartment on campus. It's 3:00 a.m.

"Be there in a minute."

"Genevieve, it's a fire alarm!"

"I know. I know."

"What's taking so long?"

"Just putting in my contacts."

"Contact lenses? You'll fry before you reach the lobby."

Daphne doesn't get it. It's a risk I am willing to take.

Contact lenses aren't only about seeing. They're about being seen—without the indignity of eyeglasses—in the right light at all hours of the day. Let Daphne head to the lobby in wire-rimmed spectacles with her neck poking out of a dressing gown and her long, bare feet shoved into slippers. I've got appearances to keep up.

• • •

My romance with contact lenses, which would later lead me astray, didn't end after university. If anything, it deepened. I had worn contact lenses enthusiastically from the moment I could afford to buy a pair with money from my part-time job in the basement of the BiWay store. Those first lenses were tiny glass saucers that suctioned onto the front of my eyes. They gave good, crisp vision but at the cost of comfort. One false move and they slid up towards my brain. One loose mohair fibre and the pain was exquisite.

No matter.

As a self-employed mediator and arbitrator, I wore contact lenses in fluorescent-lit meeting rooms and smoke-filled receptions. I wore them on planes, trains, and busses. I wore them from early morning to late at night. So what if my eyes pulsed red in the mirror or felt like they were being abraded with ultrafine sandpaper? "You must have eyes like ball bearings," a contact lens fitter once told me.

The evening I met my husband, William, I wore contact lenses. Of course.

It was a blind date, and we'd agreed to meet at 6:45 p.m. at the bank machine next to my workplace. Beforehand, I'd rinsed off my lenses in the washroom down the hall from my office and put them back into my eyes, hoping I'd be able to last the evening without discomfort.

I had heard about William from my friend, Donna. She'd been introduced to him as "the nicest man in Toronto," but he didn't meet her standards. "Too old," she complained. "Too tall."

"Well, give me his number," I said. I was into nice. Tall was fine too. And as for age—well, by my mother's standards I was already over the hill. She was running out of novenas and patron saints: Saint Anne, Saint Anne, get her a man.

As soon as Donna gave me the number, I telephoned William at the Labour Relations Board where he worked as a mediator. He answered the phone.

"Hello, William," I said. "You don't know me from Adam. Well, haha, I guess I should say 'Eve.' My name is Genevieve. I'm a friend of Donna's. She talked about you. You sounded like a nice person, and I'd like to meet you."

"Uh…" said William. "Sure. Sure."

"Let me take this a step further," I continued. "I have tickets to *Les Liaisons Dangereuses* next Tuesday, and I'd be pleased to have you as my guest." *Where was I getting this stuff from?*

"Uh… Sure. Sure."

But William explained he'd be flying back from a mediation in Ottawa that afternoon, so he wasn't sure what time we could meet up.

"No problem," I said. "Why don't you call me when you land and we'll take it from there. We'll catch a bite to eat before the show if that works."

William's plane touched down from Ottawa in plenty of time, and he was waiting in front of the bank machine when I stepped out of my office building that evening.

Yes, he was tall. Over six feet I guessed, with the chest and carriage of a disciplined soldier. His straight, fine hair— such as was left—was greying, and he had a neatly cropped, blondish beard. Laugh lines fanned out from the corners of his eyes.

"Genevieve Chornenki." I put out my hand.

"Pleased to meet you," he said.

We shook hands, and I felt a tiny *thunk*, as if a missing puzzle piece moved into place. Then we headed off to dinner and the play.

Fifteen months later, we were married.

• • •

Years later, William said that he found my initial handshake comical. "But you know what impressed me?" he said.

"No. What?"

"At intermission, you said, 'Excuse me. I'm going into the ladies to take out my contact lenses.' And off you went."

"So?"

"You came out wearing glasses."

"The little red ones?"

"Yeah."

"I remember those."

"And when you did that, I thought to myself, 'Wow! That's one self-confident woman.'"

"Fooled you, didn't I?"

CHAPTER 2

Repeat to end of row

....

"Is it OK for me to wear contact lenses into my pregnancy?"
I asked my optometrist. "I don't want to scratch my cornea
or anything."

I was forty years old and preferred not to add eyeglasses
to a bulging belly and greying hair. But I felt increasingly
uneasy about my reliance on contact lenses, pestered by the
prospect that they were an indulgence I would pay for later.

"When are you due?" she asked.

"March 25th, give or take. Whenever he decides."

"Ah, you're having a boy?"

"So I'm told."

"Congratulations. Let's take a look at your eyes."

The optometrist used a device to test several different
lenses in front of my eyes and posed the usual questions.
"Do you prefer this? Or this? And now which one's clearer?
This? Or this?"

I did my best to answer.

"So what do you think?" I asked when the equipment
was put away.

"A small prescription change. But let me take a look at your contacts."

I handed her the small plastic container where my contact lenses floated in saline.

"Oh, my!"

"Something wrong?"

"How old are these?"

"I dunno. Couple of years."

"Well, they're not in very good condition."

"Really?"

"Ought to be replaced."

"OK. Should I ditch the vanity then and resort to eyeglasses?"

"No need. Wear your lenses for now, but they really do need to be replaced."

"Can I wait till after the baby? Get new lenses and a new prescription then?"

"Sure," she said. "And good luck with the pregnancy."

I left the appointment with my conceit *and* my contact lenses intact. What a relief! I did not have to resort to eyeglasses to protect my eyes during the pregnancy.

Several months later, a curious black line presented itself at the edge of my vision, like a marker scrawl on a flip chart. Interesting. I was intrigued, but not alarmed. After all, in my experience, issues with my eyes were fixed by placing something in front of them. This new phenomenon would surely be the same, and in due course, I'd look into it. For the time being, I had work to do and preparations to make for an eight week maternity leave.

On April 3rd, as midnight approached, Nicholas Leo was born, weighing six and a half pounds. He had tiny flaring nostrils and spiky hair on a cone-shaped head. I'd been expelling him for over fifty-two hours, so wasn't much into examining or counting his fingers and toes. Instead, as I looked down at his tiny form, I said to William, "Holy crap! What do we do now?" Hospital staff then whisked the baby away to the nursery for a minor respiratory issue.

William floated out of the delivery room and found his way home to compose ecstatic poetry, and I was relieved to see him go. He'd been annoying me for hours with a stopwatch and nervous directives as he followed the baby's heart rate on the monitor. "Uh oh. The rate just dropped. Deep breath. Deep breath. Deep breath. Good, good, good."

Now, with Nicholas out and breathing independently, the only things on my mind were solitude and sleep, in that order. Back in the ward, as I settled into bed, the night nurse lifted my nightgown. "Oooh," she said. "Those hemorrhoids sure do look angry."

• • •

Hemorrhoids weren't my only souvenir from the delivery room. Bleary vision was another. The black line like a marker scrawl? Within days, it was joined by an elusive distortion and restricted vision that I struggled to pin down or describe. "It's like there's Vaseline on my eye," I complained to William. Or, signalling with my hands, "It's as if I'm wearing horse blinkers."

Unlike a hangnail, heel blister, or, let's say, a shredded perineum that results in definite, localized discomfort, the issue with my vision lacked both sensation and location. Nothing in the vicinity of my eyes hurt, and I had trouble pinpointing where or how things were wrong.

It never occurred to me to report my vision to my obstetrician or to anyone else. Instead, like a knitter trying to produce luscious fabric from binder twine, I kept knitting gauge swatches, varying my needle size but reproducing the same pattern—the something-in-front-of-the-eye stitch. Perhaps the problem was the eyeglasses that I was wearing more frequently. Sitting further from my eyeballs than contact lenses, they never did produce crisp vision. Or maybe they were scratched. But polishing them didn't help, so...? I had permission to wear contact lenses while pregnant, meaning the problem couldn't be surface eye damage. No. Not that. Most likely the prescription for both my eyeglasses and my contact lenses was out of date and needed to be updated. Yes. That must be it. Should see the optometrist again soon.

Good luck with that.

I was now employed full time—by Nicholas, whose demands were constant, ever present and non-negotiable. The way he assigned my nursing shifts was erratic and unreliable.

    2:40 to 3:05 a.m.
    6:00 to 6:30 a.m.
    8:30 to 9:00 a.m.
    9:40 to 9:50 a.m.

11:40 a.m. to 12:20 p.m.

2:35 to 3:05 p.m. (one side only)

3:35 to 4:35 p.m. (other side)

7:05 to 7:45 p.m.

9:10 to 9:30 p.m.

9:47 to 10:40 p.m. (good, long feed)

12:00 to 12:25 a.m.

1:10 to 1:35 a.m.

5:40 to 6:30 a.m. (off and on)

8:55 to 9:35 a.m. (crying)

11:55 a.m. to 12:35 p.m.

4:00 to 4:35 p.m. (snack)

7:15 to 8:00 p.m.

11:00 to 11:30 p.m.

I could no longer go for a leisurely, solitary walk. Could not work quietly on an outstanding arbitration award. Could not be out and about generating new paid work. Could not go to the bathroom in peace. Could not fit into my clothes. And most certainly could not make an immediate eye appointment.

Eight weeks after Nicholas was born, when my maternity leave was at an end, I finally visited my optometrist. My symptoms had not abated and I had plenty of practice describing them.

"Something's up with my eyes," I said. "Have I scratched my cornea?"

I explained about the black, wavy line and the fuzziness, and how polishing my eyeglasses had no effect.

"It's as if there's Vaseline over my eye," I repeated, "and I feel as if I'm wearing blinkers, like a racehorse." I put my hands to my temples.

"What you're describing is the aura of a migraine sufferer," the optometrist told me. "Just a little more astigmatism and a small adjustment to your prescription."

"I don't get migraines," I said. "Never have."

But the optometrist was the expert, and she'd been right on other occasions. Like the time she figured out that an ophthalmologist had given me an incorrect lens prescription. So, I shrugged off her migraine comment and revelled in her absolution: I hadn't damaged my eyes after all! A prescription change? A bit more astigmatism? Wonderful. Bring on the new contact lenses and make them disposable ones this time—filled with water and jelly-like.

I placed my order and looked forward to the end of distorted vision.

CHAPTER 3

Light. At night.

. . . .

My new contacts, the disposable ones, disappointed me. They flipped inside out, so I couldn't tell the right lens from the left one, and they had a gummy feel when pressed onto my eyeballs. More importantly, they didn't produce the pre-pregnancy eyesight I expected.

Still searching for a return to normal vision, I went back to my original contact lens fitter and ordered the rigid kind of lenses I'd worn for years. As soon as his office telephoned that my order was in, I bounded out the door, leaving three-month-old Nicholas in William's care.

"Oh, damn!" I said when I put the rigid lenses into my eyes. "They're not making any difference."

"What do you mean?"

The contact lens fitter listened carefully to my litany— *like wearing blinkers, distortion, clear if I look straight on.*

"You can put anything you like in front of your eye," he said, "but it won't make a difference if there's something wrong with the eye itself."

Something wrong with the eye itself? *That* thought had never occurred to me. Nor did it linger. It buzzed away like a bee done with a bergamot flower.

"Do you have an ophthalmologist?" he asked. "Not an optometrist. A medical doctor who specializes in eyes?"

"No, I don't."

"Then let me refer you to one."

Up to this point, I'd never paid attention to what sort of professional looked after my eyes. Of course, I had periodic eye exams where my pupils were enlarged with chemical drops and I'd sit in the waiting room reading until the magazine text disintegrated. But those appointments were just to find out whether I needed stronger lenses. The health of my eyeballs or the fact that they might be part of a complex neurological system never entered my head. Nor was I discriminating about the person who attended to my eyes. Optician, optometrist, ophthalmologist. Whatever.

• • •

In the two-week period while I waited to see the ophthalmologist, my eyes produced more wonders. A new black line. This one thick and straight. On the left. A clear, bright centre stage with an indistinct side show: sharp images when I looked straight on, distorted ones if I looked off-centre. And sprays of light—at night. Light. At night. It was so improbable as to be dubious. "That's funny. I just saw light," I said to myself. "But it's dark in here and my eyes were definitely closed."

My sense of balance and coordination started to slip, too, and my clumsiness embarrassed me. While walking with colleagues at a conference, I missed the edge of the sidewalk and toppled over.

. . .

The ophthalmologist was a young professional whom I mistook for a peer. "I think I have a detached retina," I offered as soon as I met him.

"Don't be ridiculous," he replied.

Earlier in the day, I had been teaching mediation with Judi, who was once a nurse in an eye clinic. When I complained about my eyesight and repeated my litany to her, she performed a series of impromptu tests, wiggling her fingers in front of my face and moving them off to the side.

"Can you see this?

"Yes."

"How about this?"

"Not on that side."

"And this?"

"Nope."

Judi knew that I'd be going to the ophthalmologist after class. "I think," she concluded, "that you have a detached retina." Her primary clue was my restricted peripheral vision—the horse blinkers!—but there was nothing in her voice or face that conveyed alarm, and I'd never heard of a detached retina before. "See what he thinks," she added.

Twenty minutes into my appointment, having dilated my pupils, the ophthalmologist bent forward to examine my left eye.

"Young lady," he said abruptly, "you have an ophthalmic emergency. Do you prefer St. Michael's Hospital or Sunnybrook?'"

CHAPTER 4

Urgent!

. . . .

"William!" I blubbered into the phone. "My eye...emergency...on my way to St. Mike's. Now!"

Panic and sweat. A thumping heart. Fear with no vocabulary or syntax. A vortex about to swallow me.

The air was wet and humid. Rain dotted the outside of my eyeglasses and steam obscured the inside. I stumbled down the stairs to the subway. What was to become of me?

I made my way to the eye clinic on the hospital's seventh floor. Somehow. But—God, no! The place was abandoned. No one was there to greet me. The reception desk sat bare, flat, unmanned. Empty seats formed sad and silent rows in the waiting area, and industrial-looking equipment stood sentry in vacant examining rooms. The ophthalmologist was to have called ahead, so where was everyone?

I strode down the hallway, intense, insistent on finding care. This was urgent. Urgent. With my flint grey suit, hosiery, pumps, and briefcase, I meant business.

Finally, a human being.

"I have an ophthalmic emergency," I blurted. "I need attention!"

"May I know your name?"

Did he not get it?

"I'm Genevieve Chornenki," I said. "Don't you have my name? He said he would call ahead."

"No need to worry. We'll take care of you." The resident's voice was steady and calm. "Let's have a look." He gestured me into an examining room, his movements spare and soothing. I deposited my briefcase on the floor and climbed up into an examining chair that had oversized, padded armrests. When I was seated, the resident shone a beam of light into my left eye and carefully examined it. The pupil was still dilated from the ophthalmologist's office.

"Wow!" he said. "Oh, I beg your pardon…"

Without thinking, I laughed. Momentary merriment.

Another man entered the room and introduced himself. He was the retinal surgeon, the person in charge. His dark-framed glasses and intense manner gave him an air of authority that was contradicted by his goatee and the little tummy pushing out his lab coat.

"You just had a baby?" he asked. He was reading from something.

"Three months ago. Yeah."

"Congratulations. I have one of those at home, too. And, you look fantastic."

"Thank you," I said.

Then the surgeon repeated the resident's actions, examining my eye with the same care and gentleness. Nothing registered on his face.

"The retina in your left eye," he finally said, "it's lifting off. Kind of like water underneath cellophane."

"Water under cellophane," I repeated. "Not good?"

"Not good at all," he said. "We'll try to reattach it."

Try? Is no try. Is only do or not do.

"Try how?"

"With surgery."

"Surgery?"

"First thing in the morning. Now, let's get you admitted to the ward."

...

As I sat in a reception area waiting for the admissions process to be completed, William arrived. He wore jeans and the blue-and-white-striped shirt he had bought shortly after we met. Nicholas, asleep, was strapped to his chest in a hand-me-down baby carrier. On his shoulder William balanced a bulging diaper bag, in his hand was my suitcase.

"Phew!" His lips brushed my forehead. "This was tough to do on transit. Glad we found you."

I nodded.

"Did you remember to bring my housecoat?" I asked.

"Of course."

We sat together in silence, but the air was fraught, charged. Despite William's warm and steady hand on mine, I was on edge. When would they call my name? What for? What next? And what about the partially weaned baby, Nicholas? I hadn't made it home in time to nurse him that afternoon, and any minute he would wake up and demand to be fed. I would have to respond. Immediately. But what if he roused just as they called my name? Where could I nurse? Anxiously, I looked around. Other people shared the waiting area, so privacy was out of the question. What to do? Divergent demands magnified by anxiety distressed and distracted me.

"Dammit. I need privacy."

I got up to scout an isolated spot where Nicholas and I could be alone. Eventually, I found a single-user washroom, but it was no help. When I took the wakened baby inside and unbuttoned my blouse, I remained agitated. My mind, a first-time skater, careened around the rink and bounced off the boards. What if someone else needed the washroom? What if we weren't done yet? What if they pounded on the door? It was all too much.

• • •

That evening when I was alone in my hospital bed, the retinal surgeon visited. I wrapped a fleece blanket around my waist and got up to listen to him.

"I need you to sign this consent form," he said.

"Sure. Got a pen?"

"Let me tell you what's on it first."

"Go ahead."

The surgeon spoke, but I heard only Charlie Brown's teacher: "Wah. Wah."

Sounds. Words. Good intentions. But meaning? Implications? I processed little of what I was told.

"What's the alternative?" I asked when the surgeon was done.

"There is none," he replied.

. . .

Early the next morning in one of my last acts before surgery, I furiously pumped breast milk with the curtain pulled around my bed. Through the fabric, I heard the orderlies shuffling about, waiting impatiently to wheel me away. "She's a nursing mom," the nurse explained. "Trying to express milk before the operation."

She poked her head inside the curtain. "Done yet?"

"Not quite."

"Finish quickly. They're waiting to take you to OR."

William was to carry my breast milk home. Once I went under the knife, he and Nicholas would be on their own.

The father–son survival camp was not as impromptu or dire as it might sound, however. William had already assumed the role of primary caregiver, taking over when my paltry eight weeks off work ended. He would continue during a nine-month leave from his job as a labour relations officer.

William had described his intended sabbatical about a month after we met while we strolled a muddy path along the Rouge River. Beside us the river ran, steady and silent, and on its banks last year's grasses drooped, pale and helpless, resigned to the green shoots that were pushing up from underneath and would soon overtake them. It was morning and very quiet. Early spring with that warm, fecund smell rising from the ground.

We'd been trading stories about trips we'd taken.

"In a couple of years I'm going to really travel," William said. "I'm going on self-funded leave for the better part of a year."

"What's that?" I'd never heard of self-funded leave.

"Time off my job."

"*Paid* time off?"

"Well, paid with my own money."

"How does that work?"

"Right now, I'm living on sixty percent of my salary, and every payday money gets set aside for the future."

"Wow," I said, hoping not to convey envy at the mere thought of a salary. "Going somewhere special?"

"Around the world," William said. "Probably starting in Asia. I'd love to go back to China. It's changing so quickly."

He was excited about exploring new places, going solo, being carefree.

"You don't mind travelling alone?" I asked.

"Not a bit. This is something I've wanted to do for a long time. Really looking forward to it."

Little did he know...

• • •

My retinal surgery lasted four hours. William, with Nicholas strapped to his chest, paced the hospital hallways until the surgeon came to tell him that the operation was over.

Three days later, I was discharged from the hospital, clutching at William like a World War I casualty and wearing a patch and shield over my left eye. The surgeon instructed me to stay prone on my left side for two weeks. Among other things, a gas bubble inside my eyeball had to dissipate. Lifting anything, including the baby, was out of the question.

CHAPTER 5

What just happened?
....

When the examining resident blurted out, "Wow!" his lapse was excusable. He was looking at a GRT, "giant retinal tear," and he'd likely never seen one outside a textbook.

For at least three or four months—and unbeknownst to me—the light-sensitive layers at the back of my left eye had been pulling away in the vicinity of my nose, and the damaged area was the one that processed images from the left side of my body. Hence, when my colleague Judi wiggled her fingers on the left, I couldn't see them. I was still able to see clearly if I looked straight ahead because—thanks be to God—the central portion of my retina, the fovea, had not yet pulled away.

At some point, a rip or opening in the retinal layers had allowed internal fluids to seep underneath and lift them. The surgeon used the image of water under cellophane to explain what went on. There are no pain fibres in the retina, so my sight-threatening condition progressed painlessly, and because normal vision integrates inputs from both eyes, I could not identify where the problem was coming from.

By the time a competent ophthalmic examination was performed on me and the problem diagnosed, my detachment had become "giant." But how big was big? Picture the face of an analog clock where each number represents five minutes. A "giant tear" covers more than fifteen minutes— one quarter of the clock. The rent in my retina covered twenty minutes, from eight o'clock to midnight.

During my four-hour surgery, while I was—mercifully—unconscious and inert, ferocious things were done to my left eye, things I understood only years later with the benefit of the internet and a copy of the surgeon's notes.

First, a 360-degree circle was cut into the white of my eye together with the clear, thin membrane that covers it. The tissue was quartered and held back with black silk sutures. A silicon bandage, which would ultimately serve as a permanent sort of tourniquet, was wrapped around the eyeball. The back chamber was emptied of its gelatinous fluid. Then a chemical was poured in to stabilize the retina and displace the liquid underneath the detached layers. This move "flattened out the retina very nicely," according to the operative notes. The silicon bandage was tightened. Seven hundred and seventy-six laser burns were applied. The eyeball was washed out with a sterile cleaning solution. Expandable gas was injected into the back chamber to keep the retina in place while it re-adhered. Finally, the white of my eye was closed with eight synthetic sutures.

· · ·

Recovering from childbirth was easier than recovering from retinal surgery. Childbirth was physical; once previously occupied territory was reclaimed, specific body parts, like engorged breasts, made themselves known and cried for relief. But retinal surgery involved a different sort of invasion. Physical, yes—because scalpels, probes, fingers, and stitches had entered my eyeball—but also psychic. Something to do with the mind. Or the brain. Or both.

In the days following my surgery, the external, physical world constricted, and I turned in on myself. I was a tapeworm larva inside a cyst, isolated and self-absorbed. I was engulfed in a torpor from which I emerged only in response to animal needs and sensations, like the throbbing of my ear under constant pressure from my lying on my left side. I was incapable of attending to the outside world, baby or no baby. I slept through the night, woke briefly in the morning, and drifted off again as soon as I possibly could. Occasionally, I had violent, anaesthetic-induced dreams.

William roused me several times a day to administer eye drops. I hoisted myself up on my elbow and turned my face upwards as best I could. My left eye—swollen, red, and oozing God knows what—refused to stay open, so William had to pry my eyelids apart with one hand and manipulate the various dropper bottles with the other. The drops splashed about and ran down my cheek.

Light provoked me, too. It invaded the area behind my eyes as soon as the sun began to rise and expanded to fill the front of my brain. Every nerve, its ending exposed, quivered, thrummed, inflated, exploded. The sensation was excruciating.

I had no words for my experiences and no capacity to interpret or understand them. I was and continued to be profoundly uninformed. Much, much later I would make it my business to change that.

CHAPTER 6

Remains of the day
....

Little by little, day by day, my strength returned and, as it did, I tested William's devotion. Our townhouse was tall and narrow, and the master bedroom where I lay was on the fourth level. Each morning William's muffled footsteps would get closer and closer as he lugged a tray up twenty-eight stairs to my bedside.

"Oomph." He put the tray on the chair next to the bed.

"Tea?"

"OK."

But the bubbling sound of liquid hitting the mug and plopping around disgusted me.

"Stop doing that! You know I hate that sound... And peanut butter on an all-dressed bagel? Seriously! Who eats such crap?"

"Sorry, dear. I know you like whole wheat, but the only day-olds were the all-dressed kind."

"Well, splurge. Buy me some fresh ones."

William also improvised a buzzer system using the portable phone so I could call when I needed him.

"Your system is the shits," I said. "I've been calling for hours, you know. Where were you? Why aren't you paying attention? Does the system even work?"

And when cooking smells, especially garlic, wafted up through the open staircase, I suddenly became energized.

"What in the hell are you cooking down there?" I yelled. "It smells totally gross."

Eventually, I was able to take the stairs down to the kitchen with its south-facing windows to join William for breakfast.

"For God's sake, close those blinds. And why are you still making that plopping sound with the tea?"

I picked up my plate and shuffled to the darkened living room, muttering profanities. When I was done, I plodded up one set of stairs and collapsed on the double bed in the spare bedroom, pulling the patchwork quilt—a present from Nicholas's Cree godfather—up over my head. There I found dark. And quiet. Soon I surrendered to sleep.

• • •

Reading for business or leisure had always been a delight, and in my briefest of maternity leaves, Nicholas accommodated my wishes. Positioned on a large, doughnut-shaped pillow that encircled my waist, he would nurse, avidly, contentedly, a man with a mission. And I would read without interruption, my feet propped on a footstool. I'd never had the luxury of such unbroken reading time; in two days I completed *Bring Me a Unicorn*, the diaries and letters of Anne Morrow Lindbergh. Sometimes I also took business calls while the baby nursed, though I quickly learned not to tell male callers what I was doing while we spoke.

Our reading-and-feeding arrangement was a companionable one that allowed each of us to satisfy our respective hunger. Periodically, I would break from my book to look down at his tiny ear that seemed to grow as he swallowed. A slow motion video of a flower unfurling or a butterfly emerging from a chrysalis. The imperceptible perceptible to me.

Now, however, I was neither devouring a book nor contemplating my son's ear. Reading was a struggle. My right eye gave only flat, constrained vision. My left? It refused to stay open, and was essentially useless. But I held on to hope, hope, hope, that it would recover.

Fortunately for me, William likes to read aloud. There's a mild rasp or breathiness to his voice, and he reads steadily, without drama. Each evening he eased himself into the wing chair in the bedroom and entertained me with *Wilderness Mother*, the '90s memoir of a woman who married a homesteading hermit and lived one hundred miles from a paved road in remote British Columbia, without running water or electricity. She gave birth to two children without medical assistance.

"Read me that bit again. The suctioning bit," I begged.

"She's quite the wacko, isn't she?"

"She let her husband use a piece of garden hose?"

"Yeah."

"Gross. Who did he suction—her or the baby?"

"Both, I think."

"What a nutter. The two of them, really."

"I'll say."

CHAPTER 7

Radio station WIFM

. . . .

While William was indulging me and taking care of our four-month-old baby, his widowed mother was in the hospital in Kitchener, one hundred kilometres away. She had fallen while moving a piece of furniture down some stairs, badly breaking an arm and a leg. Her hospitalization was prolonged, and since William's brothers lived out of the country, it was he who made biweekly car trips with Nicholas to visit her. On one such trip, our car broke down on the busiest freeway in Southern Ontario. A passing police officer managed to restart the engine, but William could coax it only as far as his mother's driveway.

When my own father became disabled by a series of strokes, William tended to his bodily needs without flinching. He knows how to use a defibrillator, keeps his first aid training up to date, and carries surgical gloves and a mask in his breast pocket "just in case." He cheerfully chauffeurs me and my girlfriends to knitting weekends even though he prefers blackjack and Texas Hold 'Em to braided cables and provisional cast ons.

• • •

"Hey, William. Remember when I had that emergency operation for a detached retina when Nicholas was a baby?"

"Of course."

"And the OPP officer gave him a teddy bear when the car broke down on the way to your mother's?"

"Yup."

"So…what were you thinking then?

"Thinking?"

"Yeah, you never said."

"I had no time to think."

"OK. But now. When you look back. All that responsibility—me, Nicholas, your mother."

"Well, I think there sure was a lot going on."

"Huh. Want to know what I think?"

"Go ahead."

"I think when all that stuff was going on, you were in your element. Looking after people is right up your alley."

The laugh lines on William's eyes crease, and a big smile takes over his face. "That," he says, "would be absolutely correct."

CHAPTER 8

Nature has her way

Nicholas slept in a wicker basket on the floor of our bedroom, and his bedtime routine began around 9:30 each evening. I watched William hold that sleepy little body against his chest as he fed Nicholas by bottle, wishing it were me who could do that. For the first two weeks after surgery, I spent only fleeting moments with Nicholas resting beside me on the mattress, and these were special occasions that William took the trouble to arrange.

When I became stronger, the general injunction against lifting Nicholas grew increasingly more cruel. His cries provoked an intolerable, visceral response. I heard not cries of hunger, gas, discomfort, or exhaustion, but howls of excruciating suffering, and, unable to provide relief, shared the baby's anguish. It took conscious discipline on my part not to pick up a crying Nicholas, especially when William was not immediately there to attend to his demands.

I was also tormented by a vague but lingering unease about nursing or, more correctly, about the lack of it. We had introduced Nicholas to formula when I started back to work, but breast feeding had come to an abrupt, unplanned end with my surgery. I fretted about the consequences of the break, even while lying indolent and prone in a hospital bed. Had some essential valence been disrupted between me and my child? Would Nicholas suffer long-term consequences as a result? *What* consequences I could not say, but the lack of specificity did nothing to dampen my anxiety.

"I'm worried about the baby, William. Is he getting what he needs?"

"I know you're worried. But do you have any idea how much that child eats?"

"Not really."

"Believe me, you have nothing to worry about."

"But what if—"

"Stop. I'm telling you. Vast quantities of formula disappear down his throat every day."

"Yeah, but he's missing my antibodies."

"Hardly."

"How do *you* know?"

"Because he's already had three months of breast milk. And because I'm the one that feeds him."

"What if he's just getting empty calories now?"

"That's impossible."

"Anything's possible."

"Knock it off. The kid has more than doubled his birth weight. He's fifteen pounds. That's average for boys his age."

"It's not all in the weight."

"You're not listening."

William repeated that Nicholas punctuated long, leisurely sleeps with six bottles of formula, evenly distributed
throughout the day, and topped himself up from time to
time with breast milk stored in the freezer.

"Sweetheart," he concluded, "do us all a favour. Devote
your strength to getting better."

A few days later, two of my colleagues came to the house
for a short business meeting. As they sat on the couch,
William came in carrying Nicholas.

"Now there's a real failure to thrive," said one of them.

"Most definitely," answered the other.

CHAPTER 9

Out and about
. . . .

A month after surgery, my left eye delighted me: it stayed open—fully—and it *worked*. Binocular vision regained! I thrilled to see Nicholas and William in three dimensions, the blush pink climbing roses in the backyard, the lacquer screen on the dining room wall, a pot of water set upon the stove to boil.

I downed images the way Nicholas gulped formula.

A week later, I was well enough for a Saturday morning visit to St. Lawrence Market. William, Nicholas, and I sauntered through St. James Park on our way there. I saw leaves, big and flat, forming a canopy over our heads. There had been none last time I passed by. Hadn't the branches been bare? Now, I was Rip Van Winkle. I'd only just slept, but how the world had changed.

Ever-present pigeons strutted about, cooing, pecking. They cocked their heads and puffed their chests. They wore five hundred and fifty shades of grey. Some were brindled. Some speckled auburn or opaline white. Their necks shimmered. The colours shifted, now pink, now purple, now green. On the way to my eyes, light waves bounced around, played with each other, tumbled about. Intoxicated by the display, I paused to drink it in, and William turned to watch me.

"Wow," he said. "I don't think I've ever seen you so happy."

"Happy? No. 'Happy' isn't strong enough."

At the market, vendors displayed peaches (already!), cherries, cantaloupe, summer flowers in a cacophony of colours—raucous reds, obnoxious yellows and oranges, boisterous blues, piercing pinks—bold, luminous colours that I used to turn away from.

What a pleasure to look *and to see*. Anything. Everything. If even for that moment.

CHAPTER 10

Optical anaphora
· ·

"Hello, my friend. You want to have some kebab? Very, very nice. Very, very good."

The scent of roasting meat on Istiklal Caddesi. A balding kebab man outside his restaurant. Inside, through an open window, a mountain of meat rotating on a spit. With a metre long knife, he shaved off a ribbon and dangled it in front of Nicholas who rode in his father's arms. Pudgy hands grabbed the gift. Into the mouth. Mmmm...

"Good. Very good. Yes? You want more?"

A nod. "More."

"You like it?"

"More!"

The laughing man offering kebab. The laughing boy devouring it.

"Jeez, William," I whispered, "The kid's eating a kilo of free meat. We'd better make sure we come back here to buy dinner."

We were in Istanbul with soon-to-be-two Nicholas, and I was living out a promise I'd made to myself while recovering from surgery. When I was well, we would go places to indulge the eyes. Soak up sights and sites: archeology, textiles, statues, rivers, gorges, grasslands, forests… Somehow I would find the money and make the time. Priorities had been reordered.

The previous year, Nicholas ate his first sand on a beach in southern Crete. We sat on an ancient threshing floor high up a craggy hill with sheep bells tinkling in the distance. We explored clove-scented Minoan tombs at Armeni and purchased belts on leather lane in Chania. Now, we would see people and places in Turkey.

• • •

In our Istanbul hotel room, Nicholas discovered the light switch. Up, light. Down, dark. Up, light… He stood on the sofa endlessly flicking the control, revelling in his new-found omnipotence.

"OK. That's enough. Bedtime."

We helped Nicholas into his pajamas and sang an impromptu verse about Weavus the dinosaur who had plates on her back and a tummy-tum-tum. Then William draped a towel over the lampshade.

"Hey!" I said. "Why did you do that?"

"Cut down the light."

"Obviously. But why?"

"Help him get to sleep."

"Oh, please! When my brother-in-law was a kid he could fall asleep in a room of yakking adults and a blaring television set."

"That was then. This is now."

"But it's bloody dark in here. Take that towel off."

"Won't be long."

I snapped my book shut.

"Spoken like a man with perfect vision. *I*, on the other hand, can't read a damn thing in this light."

. . .

Within six months of my retinal surgery, the vision in my left eye had become distorted, and in less than two years it plummeted to 20/200. In other words, what someone like William could see at two-hundred feet, I could see with my left eye only if I were as close as twenty feet. Increasingly, I had trouble judging distances and depth, and reading was a chore, especially in poor light.

The cause wasn't immediately obvious. Was it scarring, swelling, or—God forbid—another detachment? I had a collection of tests: a visual field test, a macular function test, and another nameless one where fluorescent dye was injected into my arm so the blood flow in the retina could be traced.

Good news. My left eye had developed a cataract. The lens that the retinal surgeon originally "saved" had been exposed to air during the first operation and became cloudy as a result. Opaque, impenetrable material now sat at the entrance to my left eye, right in my line of sight. The cataract blocked and scattered light, causing distortion and glare. Removing the clouded lens and replacing it with an artificial one would fix things. Cataract surgery was well established and safe.

Then the bad news.

"I'm afraid yours is a high-risk eyeball," the cataract surgeon said.

"Meaning?"

"There's risk of re-detachment."

"Ugh."

"So, I'll be doing this under a general anaesthetic."

"A general," I said. "Again."

"Your retinal surgeon will operate with me. He'll maintain constant pressure in your left eye. It's called an infusion line."

"I think you lost me. What do you do with the cataract? Laser it?"

"Not laser. An incision. Take it out in one piece, if I can. Then put in a man-made lens."

· · ·

Extracting the cataract and inserting an artificial lens took less time than repairing my detached retina, and I became alert within hours of the operation. My immediate concern post surgery was the intravenous needle still inserted in the back of my hand. I despise needles. It disgusted me. I wanted it out as soon as possible.

"You have to eat something first," the nurse said.

"Then bring me something. Please." Anything to get rid of the needle.

I gratefully wolfed down a sandwich. The needle was removed. Then I promptly regurgitated the sandwich.

• • •

What the surgeon didn't mention before the operation was that the incision in my eye would be closed with ten non-dissolving stitches and that those stitches would need to be clipped and pulled out at a later date—without my eye being anaesthetized.

A month after the cataract was removed, I returned to the eye clinic and plopped myself into an examining chair when my turn came. Trustingly, I turned my face up to the ophthalmic resident. Was this the first time he'd removed sutures from someone's eyeball? I didn't think to ask, and didn't yet know the maxim that medical students learn: *See one, do one, teach one.*

The resident moved in close and brought a small instrument to my eye. Then—Woah! I was a string-sealed bag of rice opened with one pull. My stomach soared into my throat. The room spun around. I wobbled and gagged.

"Do you feel vagal?" the nearby nurse asked in a solicitous voice.

Vagal. It's a word I've wanted to use in a sentence ever since.

CHAPTER 11

Anastasis

....

Time tempered the outcome of my second eye surgery. Rogue cells congregated and grew behind the artificial lens, causing an after or secondary cataract. Within two years, the sight in my left eye diminished. Again! More glare. More distortion. More trouble perceiving depth. More surgery with more risk of retinal detachment.

Fortunately, the remedy was less intrusive than my two previous operations. It did not require general anaesthetic, scalpels, or stitches. Once the problem was identified and other, more dramatic causes eliminated, the rogue cells were burned away in mere minutes with a laser.

• • •

The day after my laser procedure I stood at the second-floor window, looking into our postage-stamp backyard. A wooden birdhouse on our neighbour's wall caught my attention. Weathered and bare with an east-facing entrance hole, it shared space with a New Dawn rose bush, but no birds ever nested there. I'd studied the birdhouse many times, usually trying to discern why nesters found it inhospitable, but something about it was different now. What?

I struggled to work out the answer.

Then, an insight tiptoed up to me.

Before cataract surgery, the peak-roofed birdhouse that projected from the wall had instead been flat and lifeless. It hung like a compressed corpse, without spirit or presence. But now that the cataract had been removed and my brain received input from both eyes, the birdhouse was reanimated and robust. It had height, width, *and* depth. It was revitalized, reborn, renewed. Resurrected. Alleluia!

CHAPTER 12

Eye hath not seen

· ·

"Hey, Gen, my parents are into sponsoring operations that give people back their sight," said my friend Kimberly. "Been meaning to tell you."

"Give people back their sight?"

"Yeah. Cataract operations."

"Really?"

"A group out of Calgary, where my parents live. Twenty-five dollars per operation."

"*How* much?"

"Twenty-five dollars."

"Twenty-five? Where do I sign?"

And so, I began to fund eye surgeries in the developing world through Operation Eyesight Universal, a little-known charity dedicated to eliminating avoidable blindness. For each impossibly small donation, a thin, fibrous postcard arrived for me in the mail.

Dear Supporter,

We are happy to inform you that an Intra Ocular Lens has been implanted for

Name: Toba Beharani

Address: Sumandi

Age: 40

Sex: F

He/She has been discharged with excellent vision, thanks to your kindness and generosity.

I had dozens of cards identifying women and men who lived in places I never imagined visiting, and I treasured them more than my son treasured his Pokémon card collection. With each postcard I pictured the profound change that had taken place in the life of another human being who could once again see their world.

One day, instead of a postcard, a letter from the charity arrived in the mail. Would I like to purchase a place in the Woman's Tour and witness first-hand the eye care given by its local partners in India? The tour, limited to twenty female donors, would travel by air, rail, and bus, stopping at eye-health projects and hospitals from the slums of Delhi to the Indigenous communities of the Nilgiri Hills, then westward to the Bay of Bengal.

"What do you think, William?"

"I think you should go. The work's important to you, and the tour's a once-in-a-lifetime opportunity."

"But I'll be away almost four weeks."

"Yeah. We'll miss you."

"What about the business? I *am* the business."

"You're having a good year. Paid work will be there when you get back."

"William, it's India!"

"Another reason you should go."

I had never aspired to visit the Indian subcontinent. India to me was a pastiche of second-hand impressions: Gandhi and satyagraha. Madhur Jaffrey and "Very Spicy, Delicious Chick Peas" from page 106 of *Eastern Vegetarian Cooking*. Dominique Lapierre and Mother Teresa. Kolkata. Poverty. Hunger. Slums. Human misery.

What my mind assembled frightened me. I conjured human suffering on a scale that would overwhelm me. I imagined anguish beyond amelioration.

And yet, I knew that the letter was as much an imperative as an invitation. William was right. Supporting the work was important to me, and I had to take the opportunity to see it first-hand. No postcard, letter, photograph, book, or told tale could ever substitute for the potent immediacy of direct sight.

I wrote to the charity, enclosing a one thousand dollar cheque. Was there any chance, I asked, that the money could be used to fund eye surgeries at a facility I would visit during the tour? Yes, I was told. My contribution would be used to sponsor a "surgical eye camp" that would take place during my visit.

So, as five-year-old Nicholas lay asleep in his bed in Toronto, the tooth fairy about to visit for the first time, I was thirteen thousand kilometres away, and India was illuminating me with her diversity: a dense, Delhi neighbourhood where people produced chairs from nowhere and gestured for us to sit down. Families tugging me into their photo-graphs outside a temple. A lone man in the countryside, lifting his joined palms to the rising sun. Six kinds of flat-bread in Rajasthan, luxurious, leavened and not. Hoopoe birds on the turf. *Oop-oop, oop-oop, ooop-oop.* Textiles in every imaginable colour and pattern...

• • •

The white-washed walls of the Arogyavaram Eye Hospital in Sompeta pulsated in the morning sunlight that was, by 8:00 a.m., already insistent. Tropical plants in white pots lined the ochre walkways, and the occasional lanky palm tree offered its fronds to the sky.

Those awaiting surgery assembled in the courtyard and on the steps of the surgery, men and women with arms and legs projecting from hospital clothing, bright pink bottoms and pure white tops that replaced their sundry sarees and lungis.

Some of the people were more sight impaired than I have been at any time, and some were more sight impaired than others. Some moved about on their own. Others slowly, slowly, with help.

One man navigated with a stick, and it was obvious that he had no sight at all. He looked frightened and disoriented when staff, preparing him to enter the building, removed his stick. In that man's vulnerability I saw my father who languished in a nursing home in Canada—gentle face and small beard, pure white hair combed down on his fore-head, wholly dependent on others.

Travelling to the hospital by bus the previous day, I had seen a young man leading an elderly woman along a path that stretched down and away from a bright green field. She was without sight, and he guided her by means of her saree, the end of which was caught up in his right hand. He in front, she behind, the pair progressing slowly. Was that woman here now, I wondered, among the others?

My life was not that of these women and men. Our contexts and surroundings were different, very different. Still, I had some sense of what it was like to live with compromised eyesight. To misjudge distances, to see stairs when there were none and level ground when there were stairs. To be helpless in a darkened movie theatre, needing to hold William's hand—or shirt tail—depending on how fast he was moving. To feel unmoored in a food court with its sea of faces and where it was impossible to pick out the one I was looking for. But, unlike the man with the snow-white hair or the women being led by her saree, I had never experienced total sight loss. An accident of birth put me in a time and place where I was able to receive timely eye care whenever I needed it.

. . .

The hospital's head surgeon told us we could go into the operating theatre, two at a time.

"Only ten minutes each," he instructed.

"Ten minutes," we repeated to each other.

"No touching or questions."

"Right."

"No making noise."

"No noise."

"And when your time is over," he said, "you can watch on close circuit television in the anteroom."

When it was my turn, I stood at the head of a bed in the operating theatre and looked down at what the surgeon had just removed from his patient's eye. A dense, opaque, light-blocking piece of protein. A malevolent pearl as big as the nail on my baby finger. A piece of seemingly benign debris that now lay inert in a kidney bowl.

Holy God!

That just came from the eye of another human being? *That* was the thief that stole sight? *That* memorializes the moment when sight was restored?

I had come to India for that moment, come to witness directly another's release from blindness. I had waited with increasing anticipation as the tour made its way across the Indian subcontinent, finally arriving at this place. I had visited the Taj Mahal, seen sacred Toda temples in the Nilgiri Hills, and meandered through the monuments at Mahabalipuram, all the while impatient to observe the surgical eye camp. And now I had seen it, seen the ultimate.

But even as that image settled, another emerged, and what I saw had nothing to do with the eyes. I perceived, with an organ I cannot name, the confluence of two daily lives, the relationship between my ordinary actions and this practical outcome. I saw two people—the one standing by the kidney dish and the one supine under the sheets—

being carried along by a river. The liquid ligature curved from the operating theatre in India to my office in Canada, from the gurney in Sompeta to the desk in Toronto where I prepared invoices and, later, slit open envelopes with cheques from which my donations were made. Moving water jostled the two of us together in a fleeting exchange, then swirled us away to bob, float, and paddle in distant eddies from one day to the next.

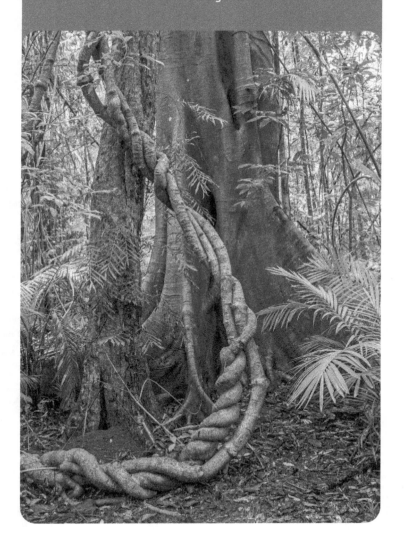

PART II

Pardon My Reach

CHAPTER 13

Wanderer, there is no road

····································

William is engrossed in online poker.

"You playing with people?"

"Nope. Hoyle's Casino. Bots."

"Then take a break and come here."

William obliges and rolls his chair to my side of the office.

"Look!" I point to my screen. "My father's lunch pail."

On Etsy, a metal rectangle with a lid like a barn roof. Thermos Brand. *Great storage box for art supplies or a funky purse!* reads the caption.

"Yeah, I remember those," says William. "You could clamp a thermos inside the lid…"

"Uh-huh. Don't know if he ever did, though."

"…and close it with those two metal clamps. Carry it with the handle on top."

"Yup."

"But this one's silver. I remember them as black."

"His was black. Put it on the kitchen counter every day after work."

"Did he save his waxed paper, too?"
"Of course."

• • •

Growing up—and even as a first-year university student studying chemistry, physics, and statistics—I didn't have the faintest idea what lawyers did. I'd never been to one and didn't know any. I rarely watched television, so hadn't seen any play-acting either. But I was pretty sure lawyers didn't carry lunch pails and *that* was compelling.

I switched out of science and into law where I soon learned that stopping for lunch during the work day, with or without a funky purse, was a luxury. Time, measured in tenths of an hour, was money, and money was generated by mastering the giant classification system at the heart of the law: *Round peg in round hole, square peg in square hole. If round, then... If square, then...*

This sorting function should have suited me, given my irrepressible instinct for organization and my fondness for categories. But there were problems.

Somehow, I'd gotten myself into civil litigation, which involved taking on other people's predicaments and arguing for their pet solution before a high-status male in a process where everything balanced on the head of a pin. Anything could happen in the tit-for-tat of a courtroom, and effective advocates must be at ease with the unpredictable nature of things. Not me. I am not and have never been spontaneous. (Ask William what happened when he dropped me off for a surprise wedding shower organized by my sister.) Nor am

I good on my feet, even without the added distraction of compromised vision.

In addition to its personal demands, the courtroom tended to inspire unsavoury human behaviours.

"Counsel, may I please have a copy of the case you just mentioned? I'm not familiar with it."

"Later."

"But we're next on the list, and you're going to use it when you stand up to argue."

"Of course. It shows how wrong your position is."

"Well, let me see it."

"When I'm good and ready."

Such was the backdrop to my reading *How to Win Friends and Influence People* by Dale Carnegie. "Be a good listener," Carnegie wrote in 1936. "Try honestly to see things from the other person's point of view. Talk in terms of the other person's interests."

What a concept!

It was Carnegie, a Missouri farm boy, not Harvard's getting-to-yes Roger Fisher, who introduced me to win–win negotiation. Once I started to recognize another person's "interests"—to talk to opposing lawyers about what they and their clients were really trying to achieve—I began to settle files, and I found brokering settlements so much less stressful than having to be someone's advocate and take their case to court.

It didn't end with Carnegie, and, before long, I had assembled a library with a leaning: *No Contest: The Case Against*

Competition by Alfie Kohn, *The Evolution of Cooperation* by Robert Axelrod, *Human Aggression* by Anthony Storr, *Autobiography: The Story of My Experiments with Truth* by Mohandas K. Gandhi, *I Am Right, You Are Wrong* by Edward de Bono.

Without mentors or models, I thirsted for alternatives, rummaged for the possible, craved inspiration.

Think and Grow Rich by Napoleon Hill, *Do What You Love, the Money Will Follow* by Marsha Sinetar, *Your Money or Your Life* by Joe Dominguez and Vicki Robin.

Eventually or, perhaps, inevitably, I stumbled on mediation with its quasi-spiritual overtones. The process of mediation, I read, begets wise and cooperative parenting by divorcing spouses, the amicable dissolution of business partnerships, robust workplaces, the peaceful end to hostage takings, and bread breaking among environmentalists and proponents of development.

If I were to become a mediator, it seemed I could shed an advocate's gown and wear my own skin. From the still point of the circle, I could help people resolve their differences constructively. I could honour logic *and* intuition. Offer indiscriminate respect to others without regard for their personal characteristics or social positions.

I took three mediation courses in two years, including one in Boulder, Colorado, at the Center for Dispute Resolution. The course instructors epitomized and emphasized human goodness, which greatly attracted me, goodness being more rare and mysterious than evil. They sketched an intoxicating landscape where, through personal discipline and constructive habits of mind, ploughshares replaced sickles, collaboration trumped top-down authority, and peacemakers were indeed blessed. Heady stuff.

I was prepared to trade my life energy for that picture. But how? I knew no one in Canada who made a living doing mediation or any other form of dispute resolution outside of the court system.

CHAPTER 14

Satyagraha
. . . .

"Margaret, I'm scared."

Before I met William, Margaret was my closest friend, the person I confided in. She knew everything about my romances, finances, family circumstances. She encouraged my exploration of mediation and fanned my idealistic embers. And when I finally decided to start my own business, Margaret was the one who helped—no, took charge of—furnishing and outfitting my office.

We were in southwestern Ontario, combing through a dusty barn in search of the antique table, burled walnut chairs, and ornate Victorian sideboard that Margaret prescribed for me. She was confident they would create the right ambiance in the room where I would help people come to terms with their differences.

"Of course you're scared," she said. "You're the anxious type."

"I could have looked for a job. With a paycheque."

"No, you couldn't. And let me tell you why. Because you're constitutionally unemployable."

"But what if I don't get any paid work—ever?"

"You will."

"How do you know?"

"Come on, Gen. It's obvious. You're Gandhi."

"Gandhi?"

"You're leading a non-violent movement. Reforming the litigation system..."

"Jeez, Meg. Gandhi didn't have two beans to rub together."

"...and we have to make sure you don't get assassinated."

• • •

The day my office officially opened and self-employment began, I felt as if I were dropping from a window forty feet above the pavement. My fingers let go of the ledge, and I went down, down, down...

The anxiety never abated, but after several years of free fall, I managed to land without smashing my talus and tibia. How to account for that? Grace, luck, accident, serendipity, mystery, or the random workings of the universe.

I graduated from mediating car accident cases to mediating out-of-province construction claims against architects and engineers. I arbitrated consumer warranty claims and shareholder disputes where I wrote gentle rulings, taking care to "judge the problem, not the people." I designed and delivered customized training for public bodies. I wrote consulting papers and advised nascent dispute resolution programs. Gave talks, volunteered on committees, taught courses at night—three while pregnant with Nicholas. It was a varied diet, to be sure, but it was regularly punctuated by bouts of scarcity and involuntary fasting.

The year I finally had to pay income tax was a joyous one, and my new field, Alternative Dispute Resolution, or ADR as it came to be known, was also beginning to attract attention, though mostly from people who wanted to do the work as opposed to pay for it.

Some time after Nicholas was born and long before the term "insecure employment" was invented, a colleague and I were on a panel at a conference where we were to speak about starting an ADR business. Steve, a much better marketer and raconteur than I, talked about a business (we all pretended it was not his) with significant bank debt and cash flow issues. Its lender required regular reports and revisions to the business plan. The partners, Steve said, were dedicated and determined, but they struggled. Thank God they had a written roadmap that illuminated their goals and milestones.

I pooh-poohed Steve's linear approach. I'd only ever done one business plan, I announced, because a friend of my brother's told me to. But once it was done, I put it in a drawer and never set eyes on it again.

I energetically endorsed the do-what-you-love-and-the-money-will-follow philosophy, and a few people in the audience nodded in agreement. When the panel concluded, several women came forward to say how much they appreciated my unconventional attitude and remarks.

Then a man approached. "Kee-rist!" he said, looking from me to Steve and back again. "You conveniently avoided the hard part—how to make any money in this damn business. Do what you love? Such crap! I tried it last year, and guess how much money I made?"

Too tempting. "How much?" I asked.

"Dick-all."

"Dick-all, meaning…?"

"Forty thousand dollars."

"Before or after expenses?"

"After."

Steve snorted, and I started to laugh.

"What's so funny?" the man wanted to know.

"Sorry," said Steve. "Too hard to explain."

CHAPTER 15

A reasonable thing to do
·····································

In my chemically induced euphoria after retinal surgery—
painkillers and residual anaesthetic—I floated about,
thinking fondly of the optometrist who had said I had a
migraine. *She'll want to know about the "giant tear," won't
she?* Her kindly face hovered, big-eyed with interest and
sympathy. *I'll tell her everything, all the details: William!
Emergency! Subway. St. Mikes. Nursing baby. Yawn. Over coffee, maybe.* Deep intake of breath. *Girl-to-girl...*

My mind drifted up, glided above the bed, and sank
back down.

*She'll move in close to listen... Mmmnn... Should I tele-
phone or drop her a note?* I cuddled the pillow, swaddled in
thought clouds.

· · ·

It faded, of course, my land of dreams, and eventually I
could see. Well enough to read a newspaper clipping on a
bulletin board in the surgeon's office while waiting for him
to examine my glued-on retina. This was before Dr. Google,
and the clipping catalogued the symptoms of a detached
retina: floaters, light, lines, loss of peripheral sight. I could

check off every box, and as I did so it began to dawn on me that retinal detachments are neither exotic nor mysterious.

"Do you think I should make a formal complaint about my optometrist?" I asked the surgeon.

"That would be a reasonable thing to do."

"I mean, that newspaper clipping on your board, signs of a detached retina…"

"They're well-established symptoms."

"And now that I know, mine seemed obvious…"

"But it takes an ophthalmic examination."

"…and I told her I never get migraines."

"Listen," the surgeon said, "a patient could tell me he sees dogs. I still have to look in his eye and ask, 'Dalmatians or spaniels?'"

"Dalmatians or spaniels. Too funny!"

"It's fundamental medicine. That's what it is."

• • •

It would be a reasonable thing to do.

I'd visited my optometrist twice. Been specific the second time—wavy line, horse blinkers. Left with a new contact lens prescription. Carried on for weeks—months— even flying and exposing my eye to pressure changes, all while my retina peeled away from the inside of my eyeball. I had since learned that the matter was straightforward: before pronouncing a migraine, the optometrist should have looked inside my left eye.

Still, I hesitated. My days of immobility and torpor, episodes of exquisite pain were in the past. Daily life resumed.

I had returned to work. William was home full time, and Nicholas grew fat and round under his care. What was there to complain about? The re-attachment was successful. I'd had a close call and my eyesight was a little compromised—I couldn't correctly identify colleagues across the room at a reception, say—but that was more inconvenience than tragedy. Future issues might emerge. In the meantime, *be here now.*

What I didn't see was that I was looking through the wrong lens: mine. I wanted to be virtuous and was preoccupied with compassion, acceptance, equanimity—all those aspects of human goodness floating in the mediation cocktail I'd been guzzling.

Then one day, I accidentally enlightened myself.

I was in Halifax, sitting on the edge of a desk and talking about mediation to people who worked for the provincial dental board and others who oversaw doctors. I wanted these regulators to understand the difference between private disputes and public ones, so they wouldn't dismiss patient complaints as mere personality clashes.

By this point I had some experience mediating public-interest disputes. I'd been part of a bold experiment for resolving patient complaints at the College of Physicians and Surgeons in my province, and I had been the first person to mediate a complaint with the doctor, college, *and* patient all taking part. I served as the outside intermediary, helping them reach a provisional settlement that would go to a discipline panel for approval.

"A fight between business partners is private," I said to the people assembled in Halifax. "The partners own it, and a mediator's job is to help them work out their own resolution. But a patient complaint, say to a dental board about a dentist, that's different. The dental board has to be involved because the dispute doesn't belong to the patient and the dentist."

The dental board's role, I explained, was to enforce professional standards, to protect other patients and the public. "That's what an oversight body is supposed to look after," I said, "the public interest..."

Before I could finish the words, an internal ping registered. I *had* to make a formal complaint to my optometrist's oversight body. This was about public protection: suppose the optometrist really didn't know how to diagnose a detached retina? Was careless? Or confused?

• • •

Eighteen months after my first surgery, I delivered a letter to the College of Optometrists. I detailed what happened to me, and asked the college to look into the matter and take appropriate steps.

As a courtesy, I sent a copy of the complaint to my optometrist along with a note of regret. "My concern relates to the public," I wrote, "and whether other patients might be at risk. After thinking a great deal, I had to conclude that it was up to the College of Optometrists to determine that, not me. I hope you will understand."

"What do you think about the note to my optometrist, William? Before I send it."

"Not wild about that last bit."

"What bit?"

"The bit about other patients and her understanding."

"What's wrong with it?"

"It's namby-pamby."

"I see. Thanks for the input."

I mailed the note as it was.

CHAPTER 16

One...two...three...surprise!

Eventually the college sent me a stern and legalistic letter. My optometrist would go through discipline as a result of my complaint. She was charged with professional misconduct: failing to dilate my pupils and look inside my eye on two occasions, failing to test my peripheral vision on one occasion, and failing to refer me to a specialist for a retinal detachment.

Time passed. Then, in November—it was already cold enough that my eyeglasses steamed up when I came in from outdoors—a male with a collegial voice telephoned me at the office.

"Ms. Chornenki, Estevan here."

"How can I help you, Mr. Estevan?"

"I'm discipline counsel for the College of Optometrists. I believe we've met professionally before."

"Not sure about that."

"Anyway, I'm calling to tell you we've agreed to settle your complaint. There won't be a hearing."

"We? Agreed?"

"Your optometrist agrees to plead guilty to professional misconduct."

"Oh!"

"With a two-month suspension. But that'll be waived if she goes through quality assurance, a very creative program. Punishment is old-fashioned. And, oh, she's also agreed to an unrecorded reprimand."

"Woah. Too fast. She's pleading guilty?"

"Yes."

"And the penalty is what?"

"Quality assurance. An office audit."

"An office audit. What is that?"

"Well—and I want you to know she's been utterly cooperative, absolutely cooperative. She's even going to pay the associated costs—"

"And the audit?"

"It's a random review of her files."

Silence. Me puzzling.

He carried on. "Her attitude and cooperation—hers and her lawyer's—they've been exemplary."

"Sorry," I said. "I'm missing something. What has looking at paper records got to do with failing to detect a detached retina on a live human being?

Silence. Then Estevan exhaling.

"Can't you make her take a basic course?" I said. "Or observe a retinal surgeon? Detect detachments in the field?"

"She may well have taken courses. I don't know. As I say, she's been most cooperative. Remediation. That's the answer, not punishment."

"I never asked for punishment."

"Listen," Estevan said before ending the call, "I've got five files like this. Not five for her. This is her first offence. But your file is nothing compared to the guy who missed a tumor."

CHAPTER 17

Calliphora vomitoria

. . . .

"Tell me again," I said. "How does randomly pulling my optometrist's records ensure competence?"

I sat at a table beside the registrar, the chief executive officer of the college. I'd requested an in-person meeting to understand the settlement Estevan had described to me over the phone. In that moment, I recognized myself as a blue bottle fly buzzing against a screen door. No doubt annoying, but I felt compelled to buzz.

"Sorry," the registrar told me. "We can't reopen the deal."

"Why not?"

"I don't think our lawyer will let us."

"Well, ask him."

He shook his head. "I can't see him agreeing to any other terms."

. . .

A few days later, the registrar called to confirm that Estevan would not add any courses to the optometrist's penalty. "But, you can come to the hearing and make a victim impact statement," he said, "provided you give us a copy of your remarks in advance. And if you do decide to come, you should understand: we'll neither support nor oppose you at the hearing."

"Sounds like the opportunity of a lifetime," I said. Then I thanked him for his call.

CHAPTER 18

Offer your light
....

When I was a child, unpaid household chores were a non-negotiable part of family life. My mother proudly told her friends and co-workers that she "believed in child labour." Dusting, sweeping, vacuuming, cleaning hardwood floors with solvent and polishing them with paste wax. Cooking, baking, doing the dishes. And laundry.

My father and brothers wore white, one hundred percent cotton shirts. These would be washed, put through the wringer, and air-dried till they crackled like Finn Crisps.

"Let's just touch up these shirts," my mother directed me.

Only there was no "us," and "touch up" grossly understated the effort required. I was to work miracles with a hot, dry iron and a few drops of water shaken from the fingers.

The registrar's offer of a victim impact statement was as insincere as my mother's ironing proposal. Neither intended for me to participate with them on an equal footing.

• • •

I told William about the registrar's offer after Nicholas was in bed.

"Sounds like a victim impact statement would give you a chance to explain what you went through," he said.

"Why make a spectacle of myself? It's not about me."

"But it could be. I mean you were a victim."

"That's not how I see myself—or want to be seen."

"But you were. A victim of her incompetence."

"Victims have no agency."

"Lighten up. What's the harm in playing along?"

"The harm is—"

"Hell, you could even have some fun with it. Work on your squinting. No. Better yet, haul out one of those black eye patches from your first surgery. And take Nicholas with you. Victim number two."

"Thanks for your continuing support, William, but no. The only prop I'm taking to the hearing is Donna, and she will be there as my lawyer."

Donna was the person who had first given me William's telephone number, but she held another important credential. She was a lawyer who, like Estevan, had experience advising professional discipline bodies.

CHAPTER 19

Call me by my true names

I wore small rectangular eyeglasses with blue titanium rims to the hearing and, on account of recent cataract surgery, had no need to rehearse my squinting. My left eye with its artificial lens generated one image, my right eye with its natural lens another, and my eyeglass prescription did not accommodate the difference. I had to hike my glasses up on my nose using my thumb and strain to see, craning my neck forward like a turtle extending its head away from its shell.

Donna preceded me into the hearing room, wearing a stark navy suit with no adornment. She is small and likes high heels. In professional contexts, she uses a cultivated, mildly imperious voice.

"Donna! What are you doing here?" Estevan knew her on sight. So did Leyburn, another lawyer—a new one—who represented the optometrist.

"I'm here representing Genevieve Chornenki in her complaint. She has some concerns about the settlement."

"Concerns?" Estevan asked. "What concerns?"

"That your negotiated penalty doesn't address the public good."

"Well, what is she looking for?"

"An educational component," said Donna. "A course in retinal detachments, for instance."

"My client has taken courses." Leyburn tossed a file onto the table behind us. "I've got details."

"Perhaps we could see your file, satisfy ourselves that the training is relevant," Donna said.

"What would you know? Are you two optometrists?"

"Let's not get excited, Mr. Leyburn." *How did Donna keep her voice so level?* "You opened and closed your file too quickly. Perhaps the registrar could be present and explain the courses to us."

In a private room, Donna and I were allowed to look at Leyburn's file. There were no courses about detached retinas. "Sexual abuse: how to protect yourself and your practice" and "Update on cornea and anterior segment" didn't count.

Donna left me by myself and went to talk to the lawyers on her own. She came back and told me she'd been able to get the optometrist to make a commitment to the college—an "undertaking," Donna called it—to take a course on retinal detachment at the University of Toronto's faculty of medicine where doctors, not optometrists, are trained.

Donna and I then went back to the hearing room and took chairs at a table behind Estevan and Leyburn. We planned to stay for the proceedings even though Donna no longer needed to say anything on my behalf; Estevan and Leyburn had agreed to include the university course in the settlement that they would present to the discipline panel.

When the hearing began, the panel chair looked around and asked, "Does counsel for the college or counsel for the member have any objection to the presence of the public in the hearing room?"

"No objection," said Estevan.

"No objection," said Leyburn.

The *public*? What about me?

"Donna! Why didn't they introduce me? Acknowledge you? Tell them, Donna! Tell them. Get up. Do it now!"

But in Donna's judgment the moment had passed. The hearing was under way. I had accomplished what I set out to do. Now it was my place to observe quietly and not be seen as a troublemaker.

At a break in the proceedings, Donna signalled the registrar. "Why wasn't Genevieve introduced to the panel?" she asked. "Please have your lawyer introduce her when we reconvene."

The hearing resumed. Estevan stood up and faced the panel. He neither gestured nor looked towards me.

"I have been instructed—no *directed*—to advise the tribunal that the complainant is here in the room," he said. His bespoke blazer, its back to my face, was explicit and effective. Effective and eclipsing. Eclipsing and obliterating. Obliterating what little remained of my equanimity.

CHAPTER 20

Hell hath no fury
....

The discipline panel had accepted Estevan's settlement, but I wasn't done yet. I knew the college had an expert's report about my eye that had prompted the optometrist to plead guilty to professional misconduct. I wanted to see that report.

"I don't need a physical copy, if that's a problem," I said to the registrar. "I'd be happy just to come in and read it."

"No. I can't let you see it *or* take it away."

"How come?"

"Because the optometrist doesn't agree."

"That makes no sense."

Donna made a formal request to the chair of the discipline panel to have the report released to me. Since it had become evidence in a public hearing, we argued that I was entitled to a copy whether as the "complainant" or as a member of the public. But Estevan and Leyburn disagreed. They pointed to a piece of legislation that, according to them, kept the report secret. So, once again, Donna and I met the lawyers in a hearing room at the college for a formal proceeding.

The room was hot and stuffy that day, but Donna and I were moved to the front of the class. We had our own table in the same row as Estevan and Leyburn (our table wiggled), and I had a "Ms. Chornenki" place card. To the right of the presiding chair was a court reporter, absent at the December hearing, with a stenomask and a pile of blank tapes, twelve high. To the chair's left was a special table for Malus, a third lawyer whose exclusive role was to give advice to the chair.

So many lawyers spending so much energy obstructing my simple request. I guessed that together they cost about $1,500 per hour. Expensive bricklayers.

After a morning's worth of legal argument, the chair turned down my request. Being the patient who lodged a complaint was not enough to allow me to see the report, he said. Even though the hearing had been a public one, if I wanted the report I should have asked to become an official participant, a "party," at that time. I was at fault for failing to follow that procedure and, as a result, could see the report only if the optometrist were to agree, which she did not.

· · ·

"How did things go at the college today?" William asked as he came through the front door with Nicholas who had, by then, graduated to the preschool room at daycare.

"Reminded me of bagging spruce sperm," I said.

"What?" He put down his briefcase and helped Nicholas out of his jacket.

"Bagging spruce sperm. As a summer student. Ever tell you about that?"

"Can't say you did." He sensed he'd better listen.

"First you locate a spruce tree. Helps to know the difference between spruce and pine."

"I do."

"Good. Then you identify the staminate flowers, the male ones, on said spruce tree. Male flowers look like miniature members and tend to be purplish when they're immature. Quite suggestive, really."

"Uh…" He glanced at Nicholas who was taking it all in. "OK."

"Then you take a bag, a specialized one with a little plastic window in it…"

"You're using a bag because…?"

"Collecting pollen to breed a better spruce tree. Think of it as arboreal insemination. Anyway, then you insert the bag over the spruce branch so you capture the flowers, making sure you don't push the branch too far into the bag to allow for growth, and you tie the bag firmly and correctly, so contaminants don't enter at a later date."

"A pretty obscure procedure," William said when I finished. "Who even knew spruce trees had flowers?"

"Exactly. And that sums up my day."

CHAPTER 21

None so blind
. . . .

I have dinner with Cheryl when my wrangling with the regulator is over. We are co-teaching in her home town and meet in the Hilton's dining room—it could be anywhere, really—cotton polyester napkins on the tables and grilled salmon with steamed vegetables on the menu. She orders tap water. I order Ontario white wine.

"So, what've you been up to?" We've been out of touch for a while, but Cheryl still knots her long hair at the nape of her neck and wears a fringe across her forehead.

"Let me tell you!" I say. "I complained about an optometrist and the process sucked."

Before Cheryl can blink, I'm off and running. Detached retina. New baby. Moral obligation. Public interest. Formal complaint. I slow my pace when I get to the personal slights so I can embroider carefully and highlight them with shiny threads.

"Get this. The lawyer for the college refused to use my name. Flat out refused. 'I've been instructed—no directed—to say the *complainant* is in the room.' That's how he put it."

Cheryl is a mediator and life coach as well as an established dispute resolution trainer. She developed "Ten Prescriptions for Peace" and her first prescription is that people must feel understood before they can understand.

As I speak, she keeps her eyes on me, makes non-committal but encouraging noises, and refrains from inserting her own solutions. She doesn't touch her water glass or reach for the menu. Her attention is gratifying.

When I finish, Cheryl sits back and looks me full in the face. "Of course, you started it."

Hey, wait a minute. *I* started it?

"I see exactly how it went," Cheryl continues. "You insulted Estevan."

"Bugger Estevan."

"No. You attacked his self-esteem. Challenged his competence. You, of all people, should see that."

No. I didn't see. Nor did I want to.

"I'm not sure you understand," I say. "I had experience with alternatives. I was the first person in Ontario to mediate a patient complaint about a doctor, and the patient was at the table. Got to talk. Have his say. Was accorded dignity, respect."

"That's your ideal?"

"Of course."

"And Estevan would know that, how?"

"He would have known if he'd thought outside the box for even an instant."

"Interesting notion," says Cheryl. "Who was in what box?"

Cheryl tells me, without ornamentation, that I saw things clearly only because I was looking down a narrow tube. Actually, I think she called it a roll of toilet paper.

"Surgery or no surgery, you still wear horse blinkers," she says. "People have feelings and Estevan was people. You called him incompetent."

"But I didn't," I protest. "Incompetent never crossed my mind or my lips. It never even occurred to me. I never intended…"

"Not in so many words," says Cheryl.

• • •

When dinner is over I bolt. Alone in my hotel room, I call William. "Cheryl blames me. Said I started things with Estevan."

"Uh-huh." I hadn't even asked how his day went.

"Hurt his feelings."

"Uh-huh."

"Embarrassed him."

"I expect you did."

"Well that was his interpretation, not mine." Through the phone I hear little puffs of air. Tell me he's not laughing.

"Sweetheart, it's like Brahma."

"What?"

"The fourth face."

• • •

Brahma. In a large, lavish building in India, more gallery than museum, a guide escorted we woman who were touring India and visiting eye care facilities. He pointed out significant items as we passed through each room and eventually stopped before an oversized image on the wall. "Here you will see Brahma," he said, "with three faces—one, two, three."

The icon pleased me. Three identical faces, serene, with dark mysterious eyes. One face looking left. One looking right. One straight ahead. I instinctively drew a correspondence with the Christian Trinity: three aspects of the divine, three facets of a gemstone radiating from a still point in all directions. Metaphor. Lovely.

But the guide had more to teach me. "Now the fourth face," he said. "The fourth face is implied."

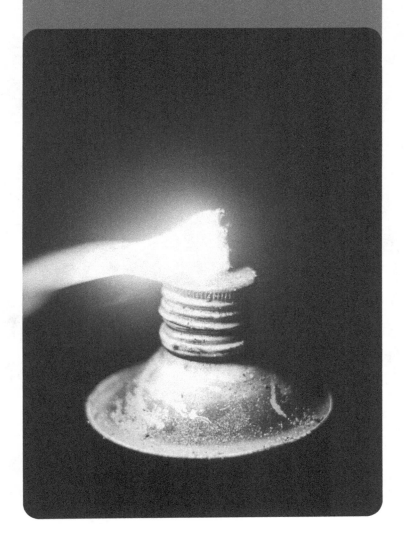

PART III

Mad Scientist

CHAPTER 22

And then...
. . . .

Time trips, tumbles, travels. Takes me to now.

Nicholas, the baby abruptly weaned by his mother's emergency surgery? The one whose maternal deprivation would mark him for life? Now a twenty-something, six-foot-two-inch man. Myopic like his mother. A doctor doing a residency in internal medicine. Not interested in ophthalmology.

William, the devoted husband who lugged a tea tray up twenty-eight stairs each morning? The one who spread peanut butter on an all-dressed bagel? Still lavish with his care and attention. Ready as his son's personal valet and my unpaid chauffeur whenever called upon.

Me, the patient? Reconstructing my days as Don Quixote, an earnest but ridiculous figure charging about to right the world's wrongs. Surrounded by stacks of paper that smother my desk and spill onto the floor: scraps covered in pencil scrawls, photocopied medical records with illegible writing, printouts of internet searches, and the textbooks borrowed from the library or retrieved from Nicholas's bedroom.

So much changed since my first eye surgery. Information once exclusive to experts or discoverable only by chance—like the newspaper clipping on my retinal surgeon's wall—is now freely and copiously available on the internet, which defines mysterious terms, points me to videos, and locates articles. And I study my findings on a twenty-seven-inch monitor.

So, I indulge. Like an avid knitter at a fibre festival, I stuff yarn into my shopping bags without regard for colour, texture, or fibre content. Who knows whether I'll knit them separately, serially, or in combination? The sundry skeins build up my stash.

CHAPTER 23

Ambitions

. . . .

"What are you up to these days?" Helen asks. She carries a pot of soup to her kitchen counter where I'm sitting and starts to ladle it into porcelain bowls.

"I'm researching," I say.

We've known each other for decades. Helen is a friend, gentle but firm. She can tell me things I'd rather not hear. "Lay off your siblings," she once said. "They know where your mother lives. Either they visit her or they don't."

Now she looks up. "Researching?"

"Trying to figure out how eyesight works, so I can put it in plain English. For a book I'm working on." Suddenly I feel foolish, exposed.

"Anybody helping you?"

"Nope. Just the internet."

"You and and Dr. Google, eh?"

"Yeah, but don't forget, I was a science student in under-grad."

Helen passes me a bowl. Carrots and cabbage float in a thin liquid. "You'll have to add your own salt."

"Anyway," I continue, "I'm very committed. First I'll teach myself. Then I'll lay it out for others. Like, how do I see this spoon and know it's moving?"

"Because you're waving it around?"

"Very funny. But what's going on *inside*? That's what I'm after. We see with our brains, not our eyes."

"Not sure I knew that."

"Most people don't."

I try the soup. It definitely needs seasoning, but I crave Helen's approval more than I crave salt.

"There's more," I say. "The retina forms from fetal brain tissue, so it's actually part of the central nervous system."

"Who knew?"

"That's my point. People think the eye's a camera, but they're wrong. What it does is convert energy. Changes it from light into nerve impulses."

"Kind of like $E=MC^2$?"

"Yeah, but more complicated."

"Hard to imagine."

"The real thorny part is how the impulses get put back together. What I mean is, how we actually see."

"See or *perceive*?"

"See. Perceive.Whatever."

"But, Gen. Isn't that like asking, 'What's the nature of consciousness?' or 'What's the brain and what's the mind?'"

"So, what if it is?"

"Well, then you're into neuroscience. That's very complicated. No offence, Gen, but you don't have the credentials."

"Who cares? I'm smart. I studied science. I'm diligent and persistent."

"Good luck with that then."

CHAPTER 24

How-are-you-I-am-fine
....

"William, there's a box in the store room marked 'Prague Goblets.'"

"Is there?"

"Yeah. But we've never been to Prague. Not together, anyway. I think it should say 'Budapest.'"

"Budapest?"

"Where we got our water goblets. Remember?"

"Right."

"But those are in the china cabinet. So, why is there a box for them in the store room?"

"No idea. I'll take a look when I have a minute."

At dinner, William breaks the news to me.

"That 'Prague' box you asked about?"

"What about it?"

"It doesn't say 'Prague Goblets.'"

"Really?"

"It says 'Fragile. Glass.'"

"Seriously?"

• • •

How *is* my eyesight? I treat the question like a greeting, "How are things?" "Fine," I say. Or, "Not bad." Or, "Pretty good." The correct answer is, "It's complicated."

My right eye is a wonder. In good light and without corrective lenses, it lets me do close-up work. I can thread a needle, lift the horizontal strand between two stitches to make an increase in my knitting, scan red lentils for stones and random seeds. Without the benefit of a jeweller's loop, I can read a jewellery maker's mark inside an antique silver bracelet. Look at other people's pictures or read texts on a cell phone if it's close to my face. Tweeze my right eyebrow, but not my left because its artificial lens prevents it from working at close range, and, no, magnification does not make a difference.

I have full range of vision. Left to right. Top to bottom. No more horse blinkers.

I quickly detect motion—we all do—which allows me to spot coyotes in the Mount Pleasant Cemetery, and my acute sensitivity to noise helps me locate and identify a ruby-crowned kinglet raucously singing in a budding gingko tree. When I'm out hiking, I need only scan my surroundings to predict the presence of rattlesnake plantain and nodding ladies' tresses.

But, there is a significant differential between my right eye and my left one, and each requires a different optical correction. The left eye needs extra help to compensate for astigmatism and to alleviate double vision, and its retina has an added layer of tissue that, fortunately, doesn't cover the tiny pit in the centre where cone cells detect colour and give the sharpest vision.

I can see the extra layer on the grainy retinal picture that I bring home after my routine retinal scan and eye examination, an examination conducted by—yes—an *optometrist* that I found through a reliable source. My current optometrist is serene, gentle, and very, very thorough. She needs no supplementary retinal training, having worked with neuro-ophthalmologists and retinal specialists during her residency. She has my full confidence.

I bring a copy of my retinal scan home and try to make sense of it. The optometrist pointed out the extra tissue caused by my retinal surgery, but despite her patient explanation, I still count more layers and labels than I saw in Nicholas's anatomy textbook.

"What does 'epi' mean, Nicholas?"

"'Epi?'"

"Yeah, as in 'epiretinal membrane.' On my scan. The layer closest to the inside of my eyeball."

"Show me."

"Here."

"'Epi' means 'on top of.'"

"Ah. Makes sense."

· · ·

Distance vision? As a rule, words and objects that are not close to my nose I see as indistinct even with corrective lenses. Sure, I can read jumbo road signs:

Cochrane 613
Thunder Bay 1345
Rainy River 1774

But I get mixed up if I am presented with too much visual information, like directional arrows arranged on a sign at different angles, because I cannot process composite images quickly enough. I miss textures and details, too, and am oblivious of what most others see until someone presents me with a photograph or I look at an enlarged image—like recently, when William and I were staying in a hotel at Niagara-on-the-Lake...

"Is that Adrienne Arsenault?" I ask when The National appears on the television in our room. I stand inches from the screen.

"Yes," William says. "She's been one of the anchors since 2017."

"I know that. But look! She has crow's feet."

"Pretty normal looking to me."

"And Ian Hanomansing. He's no spring chicken, either."

"I've got news for you, Sweetheart. Neither are we."

But William doesn't appreciate the novelty of my experience: I can *see* Adrienne Arsenault's crow's feet. What normally happens is that my brain, which is obliged to merge differing inputs from each eye, dusts over images and fills in the blanks so that I take in a coherent, albeit inexact or incorrect, image—Prague Goblets. When my brain doesn't oblige, I strain forward and puzzle over what

I'm looking at—a tendency that makes me a less-than-ideal driver. *What's the name of this intersection? Did the sign really say "No Right Turn"?* Those extra seconds are why I haven't gotten behind the wheel in years and why my daily step count often exceeds seventeen thousand.

It's a matter of adapting—to the world of well-sighted folks as well as to my own environment. I take my glasses on and off dozens of times a day so I can clearly see things that are close to me. I type on a separate keyboard and use a twenty-seven-inch monitor instead of a laptop. In a classroom or at a conference, I sit as close to the front as I can in order to see the speaker and read his or her slides. I hang an old earring on the screen door so I don't accidentally walk through it on my way to check the barbeque. I risk censure by asking for paper, not electronic, documents in advance of meetings. And I just accept the fact that I'll never be able to read people's name tags or place cards no matter what size the font.

But none of these adaptations are defining features of my existence. I *see*, and sight remains my most treasured sense. It is an endless source of delight, the portal to wonder, awe, and mystery.

For years, as a means to honour my sight, I have insisted on extended time away from paid work, time away from businesses in bitter disputes or siblings fighting over their parents' estates, time away from screens and electronic devices, time to indulge in what is presented to my eyes. I immerse myself in the natural world, far from the backhoes, jack hammers, idling dump trucks, and condominium construction sites that dominate the city where I live. And when I'm away—in the Bruce Peninsula, on some small island in the North Atlantic, or hiking the Way of St. Francis—I go days, weeks even, without checking emails or listening to phone messages. There's a monetary cost to my tenacity, for sure, but I gladly pay it in order to abandon myself to unrestrained visual pleasures.

. . .

At my suggestion, William and I are spending four weeks in rural Nova Scotia. We visit the Port-Royal National Historic Site, then take a detour on the way back to our accommodation at Blomidon, lured by the prospect of a new trail near the Bay of Fundy.

William drives cautiously along a secluded side road. Our rental car skitters on loose gravel, and the way slopes steeply downward. We are alone. Second-growth forest, dry grasses, dust, ruts. No driveways or barns. No vehicles, coming or going. No other hikers.

"Maybe this wasn't such a good idea after all," I say. Any minute now an unstable man with a firearm will emerge from the bushes. I know it.

"Relax," says William.

"I mean, we don't have to do this. We've walked a lot already today." I pull out my pedometer. "Nineteen thousand five hundred steps. Not bad."

"Give it a rest."

"No, seriously."

William navigates another bend, and I see we're at the end of the road. A lone truck is parked on the left.

"What if this truck doesn't belong to a hiker?" I ask, but William is already out of the car and studying the map at the forest's edge. I scramble out and join him.

"The Bohaker Trail's a loop," he says. "Should take about an hour." He traces the map with his finger, and I see that it leads to the shore.

I'm still skittish. "OK," I say.

We enter the path and walk single file in the direction of the shore. As my eyes adjust to the trail, the deranged hunter dissipates. Late afternoon sunlight filters through slender trees and skeletal pines, softening them. Broad leaves smother the forest floor. Coltsfoot and large-leaved asters? Greedily, I scan for blooming plants, but find none.

William and I walk in silence, feet and legs moving rhythmically, the cadence broken now and then by a stone or an exposed tree root. I continue to scan the foliage, left and right.

Then, unexpectedly, the forest opens to another world.

Mist.

Nothing more.

Mist that rises, swirls, envelopes. Reaches out with languid arms and draws them back again. Beckons and beguiles.

A spectral selkie.

"Holy God!" I say.

I'm drawn forward onto a bare basalt platform where I rotate slowly, gazing about, searching. The air is animate, primordial.

Time stops, and William melts away.

The mist and I alone now. Closer. Closer. We raise our arms, one palm up, one palm down. We circle each other. Twirl gently. Round and round. Then, hands on our hearts, we orbit a silent centre. Our robes are fashioned of fog, our sashes of steam.

Where is the sea? Where the sky? Where heaven? Where earth?

. . .

The growl of a boat motor breaks the spell.

My eyes find William. I climb off the ledge and follow him to the left with slow-moving steps. A purple-fringed orchid, alone amid iris plants long past flowering, urges me on, consoles me.

"That mist," I finally say. "I wouldn't want to have missed it. Not for anything."

William laughs. "Glad I didn't turn the car around?"

CHAPTER 25

Seeing now
·················

"What do you suppose that is?" William stops and looks back over his shoulder. We're on a cinder trail that follows an old rail line and cuts through the Grand-Pré National Historic Site.

Once more: a series of yips like a coyote or dog. Descending, tumbling down.

They stop. Then come again.

A bubbling cascade of sound. Nothing I've ever heard before. Mammalian, yes, but definitely not human.

"I dunno. It's coming from that tree." I point to a tall aspen that soars above its companions, a mass of dark leathery leaves.

Something moves.

"Hey!" I grab William's arm. "There's a bird in that tree." I curl the fingers of my right hand into a tube that focuses light. "A hawk. Oh! Two of 'em."

"Get the binos."

I unzip William's backpack and pull out our pint-sized binoculars. He puts them to his eyes.

"Hell...they're eagles. Check out the white heads."

"I don't see white heads."

William passes me the binoculars. With one hand I pull off my eyeglasses. With my other I raise the binoculars. Bugger! I can't find the birds. I squint bare-eyed in their direction and try again. "No white heads," I emphasize. "Dark all over."

"White," William repeats. "Can see them with the naked eye."

Is my eyesight that bad? I check again. "Nope. Brown."

William puts his hands on my shoulders and starts to rotate my body. "On the left. Ten o'clock..."

I slap his hands away. "No! *You* look. Over here." I point. "That dead branch."

He does what I say.

"Oh! Yes! I do see a dark one...and a nest!"

A nest? With my eyeglasses on I now notice a large mess of sticks near the brown birds.

"So where are the white heads?" I ask.

William points up. "Other side of the tree."

I strain to see. Make another tube with my fingers.

"Holy God!"

White heads, all right. Two adult bald eagles, side by side on the left. On the right, two brown juveniles, one hunched near the eyrie, one facing us directly.

A fifth bird with a tail like an open fan comes down the trail. It sails atop the tree and off into the fields. A red-tailed hawk.

The adult eagles shriek. At the hawk? At us? William and I walk gingerly towards the big aspen, taking turns with the binoculars and careful not to move quickly. Something crunches under our feet. Part of a fish spine and a scattering of seagull feathers.

"Holy God!" I say.

"Any idea how many times you've said that this week?" William asks.

"Can't help it. Just pops out."

• • •

Holy God! *noun* **1** an intense present moment. **2** a frisson of immediacy. **3** a suspension of time and space. **4** an all-engrossing now taken in through the eyes.

In *The Varieties of Religious Experience*, William James observed nature's ability to arouse mystical moods. "Most of the striking cases which I have collected," he wrote, "have occurred out of doors." Indeed.

My Holy Gods, unique and personal as they may be, confer no exclusivity. For centuries, poets, novelists, and essayists have wangled words to duplicate the evocative power of nature, especially as she is experienced through the eyes. They have conjured or questioned our joy and awe at seeing. Consider Wordsworth's "steep and lofty cliffs," Rilke's "feeling that arises because petals are being touched by petals," Levertov's "every prodigy of green," Merton's "little yellow flowers that nobody notices on the edge of the road," and MacCaig's "Joseph-coated frogs amiably ambling or jumping into the air."

"Why, why do we feel (we all feel) this sweet sensation of joy?" asked Elizabeth Bishop.

Marcus, my hair stylist, goes early to a gym in Liberty Village to watch the sun rise.

"There's a treadmill facing an east window," he says. "And the sun comes up between the buildings, just so, at different times of the year. I'm taken up. I can't stop looking."

He stakes his claim to a machine with a view.

"I go early, just to be able to see that sun. It energizes me."

And then there's Janine, whom I've known since grade seven. As we walk to the Brick Works along the Don Valley Trail, she describes a dragonfly that she saw emerging from its nymph casing.

"It was just out," she says, "and its wings were open. We couldn't stop watching. Oh, my! There was moisture dripping from its tail."

She closes her eyes.

"Its wings…as we watched, they turned clear. Sparkled."

Her eyelids flutter. She smiles and takes a long pause.

"Eventually, it flew away."

I hesitate to break the spell.

"How long did it take?" I finally ask.

"An hour? More? I really don't know. Time disappeared."

Janine goes quiet again, still seeming to relish the pleasure of her unexpected witness.

"A 'Holy God' moment?" I venture.

She nods. "For sure."

CHAPTER 26

M is for mystery
······················

"I'm on the verge of figuring it all out," I tell William at breakfast.

"Good for you." His face is buried in the latest issue of *The Economist*.

"It's very complex, but I'm not deterred."

He takes a bite of his toast and resumes reading. "Great."

"I'm finding stuff that's on point," I persist. "Even about Holy Gods. A three-hundred-and-fifty-page anthology dedicated to the pleasures of the brain and a book about the neuroscience of beauty."

I am Bugs Bunny on a break from tunnelling. Cheerfully persistent. Should have made a left turn at Albuquerque, but still headed for Pismo Beach with its all-you-can-eat clams.

"Only one problem," I say. "The research is piecemeal."

William snaps the magazine shut. "And that's a problem because…?"

"Because one article points me to another. And that one points me to another and another and another. On and on it goes. I need to close things off. Stitch the bits into a quilt, cover the bed."

"But that's how scientific enquiry works," William says. "Incrementally."

"I guess so. But at some point I need to find the research that combines the bits, shows me how to go from A to B to C to D."

"You'll get there."

"You bet," I say.

I take my empty plate and mug to the kitchen counter and unplug the toaster. Then I head to the office, boot up my computer, and open a video of a neurobiologist explaining the visual system at a 2016 conference. He lists the five areas of the brain dedicated to vision and summarizes research that supports each point. I congratulate myself on being able to follow his presentation. *Too bad Helen can't see me now.* I pause periodically to take screenshots of the presenter's slides so I can go over them later.

Pay attention, I tell myself. *This review will do you good. When he's done you'll be in a position to explain eyesight and Holy Gods in simple language.*

But what I learn in ninety minutes upends months of research and overturns my basic premise. There is no A to B to C to D, no sequence of events for me to "master" and translate into plain English. No linear explanation for eyesight, pleasurable or otherwise.

Instead, there are three—three!—parallel hierarchical systems dedicated to vision, and when they receive a stimulus, they do not necessarily operate simultaneously. The presenter says that the asynchronous nature of the arrangement has profound implications for the "binding problem."

The binding problem?

The "binding problem." How the brain puts abstract signals back together to create a visual image. The biological process by which we ultimately see. That, says the neurobiologist, is a question yet to be answered.

Madonna!

The binding problem is a question yet to be answered.

The implications are profound, all right. They're devastating. This means that no matter how much I crave a straightforward, colloquial explanation of the neurology of vision—what I've been pursuing for almost two years—I'm not going to get it. It simply doesn't exist. Pismo Beach is a chimera.

The impenetrability of the binding problem is not what sobers me, however. What sobers me is that I had been told that the issue is currently insoluble. Been told more than once. Been told but dismissed the message.

But, wait! Who told me? When? How?

I scramble for my research file, paw past notes, scour through quotes transcribed from reference books.

Before long, I have my answer. I see in my notebook the words of qualified experts that I myself copied down.

"If we ever do come to understand the visual system, it will reveal how the brain, in general, operates," wrote Margaret Livingstone, professor of neurobiology at Harvard Medical School, in 2014.

"The other difficult problem, which has bothered philosophers, psychologists, and physiologists for decades if not centuries, is how the brain manages to externalize its image: to put the world back 'Out there'. It is almost as though it assembles the information and then projects it back out, but that makes no physical sense. With our present state of knowledge, it is not clear that we even know how to state the problem," wrote Michael F. Land, emeritus professor of neurobiology at the Sussex Centre for Neuroscience, in 2014.

And this. "Visual neuroscience is full of profound questions, but disappointing answers. Vision is a superpower and it remains mysterious for now," wrote Charles E. Connor, professor of neuroscience at Johns Hopkins University, in 2018.

CHAPTER 27

On certainty

·····················

Chastened, I officially end my research and surrender the conceit of educating others about how human eyesight works. Time to clean up my office.

I sort, organize, and label my research materials. *Phototransduction cascade. Evolution of the eye. Nerve impulses & energy potentials. Brain anatomy. Thalamus. Visual processing. The neuroscience of attention. The neuroscience of pleasure. The neuroscience of awe.*

I stack old diaries and journals, including a notebook that records the start and stop times of Nicholas's nursing sessions, and return them to the cupboard upstairs.

I straighten my medical records but leave pink Post-it notes poking out here and there.

I heft a large accordion file with papers from my complaint about my optometrist. Before tucking the file away, I pause to peruse its contents. Silly me. I still have my "Ms. Chornenki" place name from the college. And here's my consolidated copy of the *Regulated Health Professions Act, 1991.* Now, what's this?

A thin stack of photocopied paper stapled to a lawyer's letter with a single line of type: "Well, after all this time, here it is… Enjoy!"

The expert's report.

When I started a lawsuit asking the court to decide my entitlement to the report, Estevan and Leyburn had relented. They eventually released a copy to me, together with a $5,000 cheque to cover my legal expenses. A victory, I suppose. But when the envelope containing the report arrived at my office after two years of skirmishing, I skimmed the materials with careless indifference. The optometrist failed to look inside my eye, I said to myself. I know that. What could this add? What difference will any of this make at this point anyway? I shredded the envelope and stuffed the papers into my filing cabinet.

But now, all these years later, I am drawn to the pages and thumb through them carefully. On top, the written submission that Estevan and Leyburn gave to the discipline panel in support of their settlement. Then handwritten notes that I take to be from my optometrist's file. Next, an official college bulletin on "Standards for the Use of Mydriatics and Cycloplegics." And finally, the expert's opinion—only two pages long? Wonder what it says.

I settle back to read the stapled papers…

Hey! Wait a minute.

The optometrist recorded in her notes that she had, in fact, looked inside my eye. She used an ophthalmoscope, a tiny flashlight of sorts. At least her handwriting says so. She looked. Inside my eye. After all.

Oh! My long-standing narrative is based on a wrong premise? That she didn't look in my eye? Oh, oh, oh...

Not so fast.

I pick up the expert's report and discipline myself to read slowly and deliberately. I pretend I am an outsider with no prior knowledge of what went on. I suspend my opinions, if only for a moment.

The expert says that the optometrist looked in my eyes, *but not properly*. She failed to meet her professional standard in two ways. First, she should have used a mydriatic. I type the letters into my computer, M-Y-D-R-I... A drug that causes the pupil to dilate, thus allowing a better look at the inside of the eye. Why a mydriatic? Because when you shine a light in someone's eyes, their pupils constrict and you see a lot less through a smaller hole.

The expert says that not only should the optometrist have dilated my pupils when I came complaining of my vision after Nicholas was born, she ought to have dilated them when I came seeking absolution for contact lenses while still pregnant. I am highly myopic, meaning that I have long eyeballs, and a high degree of myopia increases the risk of retinal detachment.

There is more.

The optometrist tested how clearly I could see things, the familiar letters-on-the-chart kind of thing. What she did not do and what the expert says she should have done was test *where* I could or could not see things. She did not test my peripheral vision. The optometrist should have done what my colleague Judi did when she wiggled her fingers in front of my face and moved them off to the side, asking, "Do you see this? What about this? And what about this?"

Without doing these two basic examinations, the optometrist was in no position to make any diagnosis. She could not properly conclude that I had an ocular migraine instead of a detached retina. The two conditions share common symptoms—black lines, sprays of light, reduced or distorted vision—but my symptoms could have had other causes too, like a tumour in the tract running from my eyes to my brain. So, how had the optometrist reached any reasonable conclusion?

I cross-check with the twentieth edition of *Harrison's Principles of Internal Medicine* that I've borrowed from Nicholas. The text says that a diagnosis of retinal detachment is to be confirmed "by ophthalmoscopic examination."

• • •

A week later, I meet Donna at Starbucks in the old Britnell's bookshop on Yonge Street. Gone are her trim business suits and pumps; she arrives in walking shorts and running shoes.

I pay for Donna's coffee. Then I play Armand Gamache in a Louise Penny novel, explaining how, once I had *all* of the clues, I assembled them to reach an entirely obvious conclusion, one that exposed the magnitude of my optometrist's error.

I end with a flourish. "Spaniels or Dalmatians? Fundamental medicine. Just like the retinal surgeon said!"

Donna nods. "I've thought about that for years."

"You have?"

"Yup. We were too lenient. I don't know what ever happened to her, but a one-day course wasn't enough. We should have pushed for complete retraining."

CHAPTER 28

This is happiness
....

...the world is a continuous, restless swarming of things,
a continuous coming to light and
disappearance of ephemeral entities.
—Carlo Rovelli

On the last day of July, William and I sit at a plastic table in
our diminutive downtown yard. He occupies himself with
Puzzler's Giant Book of Sudoku 55. I work on a Fair Isle hat
from *Vogue Knitting* using Jamieson's Shetland Spindrift in
colours of *Yell Sound Blue*, *Nighthawk*, *Sand*, and *Buttermilk*.
They're the closest I'll get to Scotland since COVID-19 cur-
tailed our plans for St. Cuthbert's Way and the Holy Island
of Lindisfarne, but I'm at ease with that.

By now, I have taken in more than my fair share of
splendor through the eyes, from Old Man on His Back
Grasslands in Saskatchewan to Western Brook Pond in
Newfoundland, from the Callanish Stones on the Isle of
Harris to the Maras Salt Mines in Peru. I've had delicious,
first-hand views of artifacts once accessible to me only in
books: Artemis of Ephesus, the Gundestrup cauldron, a
five-thousand-year-old Quipu, the Belitung Shipwreck...

My neighbour's air conditioner hums on the other side of a wooden fence that divides our half pint patios. The city is hot, its air unusually dry. The plants in our outdoor containers sprawl listlessly. I should get up and water them. Instead, I drag a spare chair towards me and prop up my feet. Easier on the back.

Index finger, knit six *Yell*. Middle finger, knit four *Buttermilk*. Index finger, knit six *Yell*. Middle finger, knit four *Buttermilk*... A corona of leaves emerges from my stitches. At the end of the round when I pause to smooth them out, a flitting white butterfly catches my attention.

"That little bugger is back," I announce. "Damn cabbage butterfly. See it?"

William is concentrating, clicking his pen.

"Hope it doesn't lay eggs," I say. "Ever seen how fast their caterpillars eat through a pot of brassicas? One year they did it in the course of a morning. Start of the day, seedlings. Noon, gone. So, this year I kept an eye out and, sure enough, they showed up. They're exactly the same colour as kale stems. Same diameter, too. Perfectly camouflaged till I took off my glasses to get a better look and found them. Squashed them in a paper towel. Gross, I know, but lovely colour—parakeet green."

William writes more numbers on his grid and gives himself a thumbs up.

"You know, I can never understand what you find so interesting in that sudoku. I mean, I don't know how it works but it looks tedious. So why would you? And check out our scarlet runner beans. What's your estimate?" I continue. "Ten feet high? Twelve? There are flowers way, way up there, but where are the beans? It's bloody August tomorrow and still no beans."

My neighbour's air conditioner cuts out with a *brrr*, and as it does, a Thumbelina-like form appears, sweeps towards the carmine blossoms high off the ground, hovers—just for an instant—then rises up, and vanishes.

Was that what I think it was? Here? Among brick walls and concrete steps? In this stifling city?

"Holy God!"

"Now what?" There's an edge to William's voice, but I make no answer.

"What?" he repeats. "You've been chattering away for the last fifteen minutes and now that you have my full attention…"

"Hummingbird," I whisper. "Just now."

I can rouse myself to say no more, for something—I don't know what—has taken me elsewhere, occupied me, suffused each space and fibre, the seen and the unseen. An extravagant abundance. A satiety of a superlative sort. One that fills yet has no volume.

And in the moment—if indeed I am in space and time—there is nothing I need or want.

GRATITUDE AND ACKNOWLEDGMENTS

This book has been gestating for a long time. I wrote the first words of an eye essay years ago in a workshop with Sharon Butala, whose *Perfection of the Morning* had enchanted me. Fellow students suggested that the story of my close call with sight loss could enlighten the general public, and I remain grateful for those grains of encouragement. But writing more had to wait while William and I raised a small boy.

When I eventually returned to my eye essay, I enjoyed the support and encouragement of many people. Anne Gottlieb read instalments of a very early draft and urged me to continue. Donna Campbell, who witnessed parts of my story first-hand, tracked my progress without ever trying to influence what I wrote. Sara Wolch shared her extensive documentary-making experience, allowing me to see how I might better convey my story. Tony van Straubenzee took a lively interest in the book and emailed me for progress updates. And my four beta readers, Emily Chatten, Michelle Cho, Janine MacDonald, and Patricia Raymond took time to read and gently explain what others might (and might not) relate to.

Shaughnessy Bishop-Stall was, to his credit and my benefit, not as gentle as my beta readers. My primary editor, Shaughnessy critiqued tone and pointed out shrill or shallow segments without ever using those adjectives. He censored sentence fragments. He scrutinized verb tenses. But he was always willing to engage with me as a peer when I queried his feedback. If my writing evinces any measure of craftsmanship, it is largely attributable to Shaughnessy. I love him almost as much as I love the retina specialist who saved my left eye—and in the same way.

And speaking of retinas, I can never adequately thank those who, on more than one occasion, attended to my eyesight at the St. Michael's Hospital Eye Clinic and at the Retina Unit of the hospital's Department of Ophthalmology. I was an unexceptional patient, and I am sure they have long forgotten me, but I have not forgotten their expertise, gentleness, and compassion.

I also wish to acknowledge the Creative Writing program at the University of Toronto's School of Continuing Studies and its generous instructors, especially Kim Echlin, who taught The Scribal Art, and Marina Nemat, who taught Writing the Memoir. I entered the program versed only in informational writing where the primary goals are clarity, crispness, and accuracy, and where, as poet Mary Oliver says, words "do not ever desire to throw two shadows." What a delight to learn that a writer can play with words, can knit or embroider with them, not only to convey information but to offer readers their own personal experiences.

Last, but by no means least, I am grateful to Nicholas for permission to publish this, a story that is as personal to him as it is to me. Enough said.

And as for William—well, if you've read this far, you will understand what he has had to contend with over the years, and you will appreciate that my indebtedness to him is limitless.

NOTES AND REFERENCES

PREFACE

The quote is from *He Held Radical Light: The Art of Faith, the Faith of Art* by Christian Wiman (2018).

PART I: NOTHING IS OBVIOUS TO THE UNINFORMED

Henry Zaluski, an executive at a Toronto communications company, taught me that "nothing is obvious to the uninformed." I have yet to exhaust the applications of his saying.

CHAPTER 5: WHAT JUST HAPPENED?

Most of this chapter was recreated from the retina specialist's typewritten notes and handwritten nursing notes.

Until my diagnosis and surgery, I had never heard the terms "detached retina" or "retinal tear," and although the eye clinic at St. Michael's Hospital was always crowded with patients, I knew no one who had experienced a rent in their retina. Now, I commend "What I Can't See," Russell Smith's account of his detached retina published in *Toronto Life* in April 2012, and his e-book, *Blindsided: How Twenty Years of Writing About Booze, Drugs and Sex Ended in the Blink of an Eye.*

CHAPTER 10: OPTICAL ANAPHORA

In her 2018 memoir *Handywoman*, knit designer Kate Davies describes how a brain injury at age thirty-six put her in awe of abilities she had not previously considered. As she learned to braid her hair and to knit again, she realized that each individual function was "the most incredible kind of miracle." I wholeheartedly adopt Davies's characterization, especially in relation to eyesight.

CHAPTER 12: EYE HATH NOT SEEN

Around the world in 2020, about a billion people had some form of vision impairment that could have been prevented or treated. Over sixty-five million of them had cataracts, an easily remedied condition. See the World Health Organization's fact sheet, "Blindness and vision impairment," October 8, 2020.

Operation Eyesight Universal (www.operationeyesight. com) continues to carry out its mission to "prevent blindness and restore sight."

CHAPTER 13: WANDERER, THERE IS NO ROAD

There are many English translations of Antonio Machado's poem "Wanderer." One of my favourites is Robert Bly's translation in *The Soul Is Here for Its Own Joy* (1995).

CHAPTER 19: CALL ME BY MY TRUE NAMES

This chapter title was inspired by "Please Call Me by My True Names," one of the poems in *Call Me by My True*

Names by Thich Nhat Hahn (1999). Each reading reminds me that I am both a frog swimming in a pond and the snake that devours said frog. See Chapter 21 where my colleague Cheryl tried, unsuccessfully, to convey the same message.

CHAPTER 25: SEEING NOW

...*steep and lofty cliffs*: "Lines" by William Wordsworth in *The Norton Anthology of Poetry*, Fifth Edition, edited by Ferguson, Salter, and Stallwothy (2005).

...*feeling that arises because petals are being touched by petals*: "Bowl of Roses" by Rainer Marie Rilke in *The Essential Rilke*, selected and translated by Galway Kinnell and Hannah Liebmann (1999).

...*every prodigy of green*: "Celebration" by Denise Levertov in *The Collected Poems of Denise Levertov* (2013).

...*little yellow flowers that nobody notices on the edge of the road*: "Things in Their Identity" in Chapter 5 of *New Seeds of Contemplation* by Thomas Merton (1961).

...*Joseph-coated frogs amiably ambling or jumping into the air*: "One of the Many Days" by Norman MacCaig in *Joy: 100 Poems*, edited by Christian Wiman (2017).

...*Why, why do we feel (we all feel) this sweet sensation of joy?*: "The Moose" by Elizabeth Bishop in *Joy: 100 Poems*, edited by Christian Wiman (2017).

PART III: MAD SCIENTIST

I couldn't possibly list all of the websites, articles, videos, and books that I consulted in my vain attempts to fathom human eyesight and understand the neural mechanisms of Holy Gods.

Obstinately determined to master how the retina converts light rays to electrical signals, I spent hours online with Zachary Murphy of Ninja Nerd Science, playing and replaying his tutorial on the phototransduction cascade. Up to that point, I did not even know the verb "to transduce." Me, a former science student...

Then, after stumbling on Semir Zeki's name in a book about beauty and science, I repeatedly watched his lecture on how the brain constructs a visual image, delivered at Barcelona Cognition, Brain and Technology Summer School, 9th edition. Zeki is a professor of neuroaesthetics.

Other references that I consulted included the following:

Blumenfeld, Hal, *Neuroanatomy through Clinical Cases, Second Edition* (2010).

Burke Feldman, Edmund, *Varieties of Visual Experience: Art as Image and Idea* (1972).

Dawkins, Richard, *Climbing Mount Improbable*, Chapter 5 (1996).

Jameson, J. Larry, *Harrison's Principles of Internal Medicine, Twentieth Edition* (2018).

Kolb, Helga, "How the retina works," 28 American Scientist, Volume 91 (2003).

Land, Michael F., *The Eye: A Very Short Introduction* (2014).

Land, Michael F. and Russell D. Fernald, "The Evolution of Eyes," Annual Review of Neuroscience, 15:1–29 (1992).

Linden, David J. (editor), *Think Tank: Forty Neuroscientists Explore the Biological Roots of Human Experience* (2018).

Livingstone, Margaret, *Vision and Art: The Biology of Seeing* (2014).

Rothenberg, David, *Survival of the Beautiful: Art, Science and Evolution* (2011).

Vilis, Tutis, *My Brain Notes for Medical Students*, Chapter 2 (2017).

CHAPTER 28: THIS IS HAPPINESS

This chapter title was inspired by Niall Williams's evocative novel *This Is Happiness* (2019). The quote is from *Seven Brief Lessons on Physics* by Carlo Rovelli (2014).

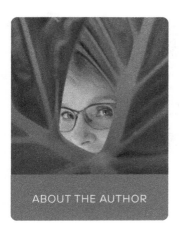

ABOUT THE AUTHOR

Genevieve Chornenki is a dispute resolution consultant and emerging writer based in Toronto, Canada. When she was in grade 4, the teacher noted on her report card, "Has excellent story-writing ability which should be encouraged as much as possible." No one in the family noticed. Nor did first prize for poetry in high school relieve her of household chores like washing dishes and sweeping the kitchen floor. Eventually, she figured out that writing is about persistence, not permission. It also helps to have something to say. Genevieve holds a Master of Laws in Alternative Dispute Resolution from Osgoode Hall Law School, a Certificate in Creative Writing from the University of Toronto, and a Certificate in Publishing from Ryerson University. Her works include *Bypass Court: A Dispute Resolution Handbook* and *When Families Start Talking*, a CBC Ideas radio documentary. Visit her at **www.genevievechornenki.com** or email her at **gac@chornenki.com**.